INTRODUCTION TO NUTRITION, EXERCISE, AND HEALTH

STUDENT STUDY GUIDE
AND
WORKBOOK

INTRODUCTION TO NUTRITION, EXERCISE, AND HEALTH

STUDENT STUDY GUIDE AND WORKBOOK

Victor L. Katch
Professor of Kinesiology
Associate Professor of
Pediatrics
The University of Michigan
Ann Arbor, Michigan

Frank I. Katch
Professor of Exercise Science
The University of Massachusetts
Amherst, Massachusetts

William D. McArdle
Professor of Physical Education
Queens College
The City University of New York
Queens, New York

PHILADELPHIA • LONDON

LEA & FEBIGER
1993

Lea & Febiger
200 Chester Field Parkway
Malvern, Pennsylvania 19355-9725
U.S.A.
(215) 251-2230

This workbook was created on an Apple Macintosh Quadra 700 with 20 MB of internal RAM and a 140 megabyte hard disk. We used System 7.01, Nisus 3.16 and Microsoft Word 5.0 word processors, and Publish It-Easy 2.19 desktop layout program. The material was printed on a Newgen 600 dpi laser printer.

PRINTED IN THE UNITED STATES OF AMERICA

Print number: 5 4 3 2 1

To our students

PREFACE

This **Study Guide and Workbook** is a resource companion to the textbook, <u>Introduction to Nutrition, Exercise, and Health.</u> Its purpose is to facilitate your understanding of the text content by focusing on key terms and concepts, and on specific questions within each chapter. The addition of test questions and crossword puzzles also should be of help.

Your **Study Guide and Workbook** is divided into three sections. Section I asks you to define key terms and concepts. These are arranged in the same order as they appear in the text, where they are highlighted in bold type. Similarly, the study questions are positioned in relation to the appropriate section that provides relevant material to answer the question. After reading the chapter and answering the key terms and questions, you'll be ready to take the sample quiz that consists of multiple choice, fill-in, and true/false questions. The answers to these questions appear in Section III.

Section II of the **Study Guide and Workbook** includes six self-assessment tests. The tests are designed to provide a realistic appraisal of your current status on important measures of nutrition, health, and fitness. Your personal health and fitness profile that emerges from these assessments should establish an objective basis to make meaningful changes in your lifestyle. We encourage you to take these tests and think about how to use the results to enhance your personal health and wellness. It is our belief that the more information you have about yourself, the better able you will be to make wise personal health and wellness decisions.

Section III includes answers to the questions and crossword puzzles, and helpful hints for studying and preparing for exams.

We are grateful to Tom Colaiezzi, Rick Perry, John Spahr, Jr., and Matt Harris of Lea & Febiger for their continued support and encouragement. We would like to express a heartfelt thank you to all of our students who took the time to provide constructive criticism and ideas. Special thanks, as always, to our wives (Heather, Kerry, and Kathy) who are becoming accustomed to papers on the floor, and our continual search for "just one more minute on the computer."

Victor L. Katch, Ann Arbor, Michigan
Frank I. Katch , Amherst, Massachusetts
William D. McArdle, Sound Beach, New York

TABLE OF CONTENTS

SECTION I

- **DEFINE KEY TERMS AND CONCEPTS**
- **STUDY QUESTIONS**
- **PRACTICE QUIZZES**
- **CROSSWORD PUZZLES**

PART 1

NUTRITION AND ENERGY FOR BIOLOGIC WORK

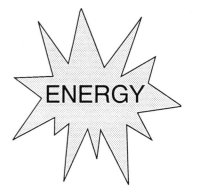

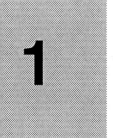

BIOLOGY AND CHEMISTRY BASICS

THE LINK TO A BETTER UNDERSTANDING OF NUTRITION, EXERCISE, AND HEALTH

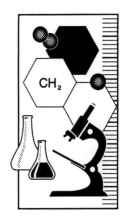

DEFINE KEY TERMS AND CONCEPTS

1. Matter

2. Inertia

3. Mass

4. Weight

5. Kilograms

6. Density

7. Elements

8. Organ systems

9. Cells

10. Plasma membrane

11. Nucleus

12. DNA

13. RNA

14. Mitochondria

15. Molecules

16. Atoms

17. Atomic nucleus

18. Protons

19. Neutrons

20. Electrons

21. Planetary model

22. Orbital model

23. Atomic number

24. Mass number

25. Ions

26. Cation

27. Anion

28. Electrolyte

29. Isotopes

30. Chemical bonds

31. Valence shell

32. Ionic bonds

33. Covalent bonding

34. Organic compounds

35. Hydrogen bonds

36. Compounds

37. Mixtures

38. Solutions

39. Suspension

40. Colloids

41. Isomers

42. Trans-fatty acids

43. Energy

44. First law of thermodynamics

45. Photosynthesis

46. Respiration

47. Biologic work

48. Mechanical work

49. Chemical work

50. Transport work

51. Potential energy

52. Kinetic energy

53. Biosynthesis

54. Enzyme

55. Substrate

56. Enzyme-substrate complex

57. Lock and key mechanism

58. Hydrolysis

59. Condensation

60. Peptide bond

61. Oxidation

62. Reduction

63. Redox reaction

64. NAD

65. FAD

66. Respiratory chain

67. Electron transport

68. Acid

69. Base

70. pH

71. Acid-forming foods

72. Alkaline-forming foods

73. Buffers

74. Acidosis

75. Alkalosis

76. Chemical buffer

77. Ventilatory buffer

78. Renal buffer

79. Diabetes

80. Homeostasis

81. Passive transport

82. Active transport

83. Simple diffusion

84. Concentration gradient

85. Facilitated diffusion

86. Osmosis

87. Osmolarity

88. Osmotic pressure

89. Isotonic

90. Hypertonic

91. Edema

92. Hypotonic

93. Filtration

94. Sodium-potassium pump

95. Coupled transport

96. Symport

97. Bulk transport

98. Exocytosis

99. Endocytosis

100. Phagocytosis

101. Pinocytosis

102. Receptor-mediated endocytosis

Matter

Describe one fundamental property of matter.

Mass

Weight

Describe the differences between mass and weight.

<u>Mass</u>

<u>Weight</u>

Density

List three factors that determine a person's body density.

1.

2.

3.

Elements

How many known elements are there? Of these, how many naturally occur in nature?

<u>Known elements</u>

<u>Naturally occurring elements</u>

Distribution of elements in the body

List the three most abundant elements in the human body.

1.

2.

3.

Cellular organization

Draw an illustration of the cellular organization of the human body.

Organ systems

List the 11 organ systems of the body.

1.   7.

2.   8.

3.   9.

4.   10.

5.   11.

6.

Cells

Draw and label a cell and its major structures.

Atoms

  Molecules

Draw and label a diagram of an atom and a molecule.

    <u>Atom</u>

    <u>Molecule</u>

Ions

What is the difference between cations and anions?

    <u>Cations</u>

    <u>Anions</u>

Isotopes

List two common isotopes and give one example of their use in nutrition research.

    <u>Isotope</u>   <u>Use</u>

      1.

      2.

Chemical bonding: forces of attraction that hold atoms together

List the three main types of chemical bonding.

1.

2.

3.

Compounds

List three different compounds and the chemical formula of each.

<u>Compound</u>   <u>Chemical Formula</u>

1.

2.

3.

Mixtures

List three types of mixtures.

1.

2.

3.

Isomer

List one isomer and give its importance.

Cis- and trans-isomers

How are trans-fatty acids formed?

Energy

How do you know when energy has been released?

The first law of thermodynamics

Give an example of the first law of thermodynamics.

Photosynthesis and respiration

Photosynthesis

List two results of the process of photosynthesis.

1.

2.

Cellular respiration

The energy released during cellular respiration is used to sustain what three forms of biologic work?

1.

2.

3.

Potential and kinetic energy

The total energy of any system consists of what two components? Give an example of each.

<u>Component</u>   <u>Example</u>

1.

2.

Enzymes

List two examples of important catalysts in the body.

1.

2.

Hydrolysis and condensation: the basis for digestion and synthesis

Hydrolysis reactions

Give two examples of hydrolysis reactions and explain why each is important.

1.

2.

Condensation reactions

Give one example of a condensation reaction.

Oxidation and reduction reactions

Give one example of a "redox" reaction during exercise.

Acid-base concentration and pH

      List two differences between an acid and a base.

         1.

         2.

Enzymes and pH

      Explain the effect of pH on enzyme function.

Buffers

      List three mechanisms that regulate the acid-base balance of the body and give one example of each.

Mechanism	Example
1.	
2.	
3.	

Factors affecting pH balance

      Describe four factors that can dramatically alter acid-base balance in the body.

         1.   3.

         2.   4.

Transport of nutrients across cell membranes

Describe two processes for transporting substances across plasma membranes.

1.

2.

Passive transport processes

List four categories of passive transport and give one characteristic of each type.

<u>Category</u>   <u>Characteristic</u>

1.

2.

3.

4.

Active transport processes

What is the role of active transport in cellular function?

Coupled transport

How does coupled transport differ from active transport?

Sodium-potassium pump

Describe the sodium-potassium pump.

Bulk transport

Outline the process of bulk transport.

PRACTICE QUIZ

MULTIPLE CHOICE

1. The following are metric units of measurement:
   a. lb, in, meters, slugs
   b. slugs, centimeters, feet, lb, kg
   c. millimeters, kg, kilometers, liters
   d. liters, pounds, m², PSI
   e. all of the above

2. All cells share these common components:
   a, plasma membrane, RNA, DNA
   b. RNA, DNA, atoms, molecules, nucleus
   c. proteins, fats, carbohydrates
   d. chromatin, membranes, cristae
   e. none of the above

3. The first law of thermodynamics states that:
   a. energy can be created from ADP synthesis
   b. energy is neither created nor destroyed, but is transformed from one form to another
   c. energy degrades whenever work is performed
   d. energy is stored in the mitochondria
   e. energy is liberated in proportion to the amount of heat gained

4. An example of a coupled redox reaction is the:
   a. reduction of hydrogen and subsequent oxidation of oxygen
   b. oxidation of hydrogen and subsequent reduction of oxygen
   c. reduction of pyruvate and oxidation of lipid
   d. oxidation of glucose and reduction of pyruvate
   e. none of the above

5. Simple diffusion, facilitated diffusion, osmosis, and filtration:
   a. are examples of active transport
   b. are examples of passive transport
   c. are examples of both active and passive transport
   d. reflect energy-producing reactions
   e. reflect energy-consuming reactions

FILL-IN

1. The body is composed of _____ organ systems.

2. _____ is formed in the cell under the direction of DNA, and is the messenger by which coded information in DNA is transmitted.

3. Na^+, Cl^-, K^+, and H^+ are examples of _____.

4. Photosynthesis is the reverse of _____.

5. Oxidation involves any process in which an atom _____ electrons with a corresponding _____ in valence.

TRUE / FALSE

1. _____ Humans are composed of 65% oxygen, 18% carbon, 10% hydrogen, and 3% nitrogen.

2. _____ Mass equals weight divided by the force of gravity.

3. _____ Three common structural characteristics of living cells are molecules, atoms, and mitochondria.

4. _____ As work increases, the transfer of energy increases so that a change occurs.

5. _____ Buffering is used to designate reactions that maximize changes in pH.

Chapter 1

ACROSS

1 Compound or process that minimizes changes in H$^+$ concentration
4 Chemical bond involving transfer of electrons between two neutral atoms
7 Synthesis of protein involves this type of chemical bond
9 One of three forms of biologic work
10 Substance that ionizes in solution to produce hydroxyl ions
11 Energy-requiring process for the transport of large molecules through cellular membranes
13 Negatively charged atomic particle
18 Fundamental material that makes up matter
20 The capacity to produce change or perform work
22 A material substance that occupies space and has mass
24 Collection of tissues joined together to perform a common function
26 Simplest unit into which matter can be divided without the release of charged particles
30 Atoms with a positive or negative electrical charge
32 Substances that ionize in solution to give off hydrogen ions
34 Form of energy that is useless for biologic work
36 An enzyme interacts with a substance much like a key fitting into this object
37 Significant drop in the pH of body fluids
38 All of the energy-requiring, life-sustaining cellular processes

DOWN

2 Hydrogen-accepting coenzyme containing riboflavin
3 The buffering system provided by the kidneys
5 Central command center of a cell
6 Nucleic acid that transmits the character of inherited traits
8 Protein catalyst
12 Metric equivalent of 2.2 pounds
14 Positively charged ion
15 Coupled reaction involving oxidation and reduction
16 Form of biologic work involving cellular growth
17 These represent the basic units of life
19 Accumulation of fluid in body tissues
21 The messenger by which coded information in DNA is transmitted
22 Quantitative measure of the inertia of an object
23 Margarine contains 17 to 25% of this type of fatty acid, butter only 7%
25 Positively charged atomic particle
27 Another name for the cell membrane
28 Substance formed from two or more different elements
29 Model of atomic structure where electrons move randomly about the nucleus
31 The law of thermodynamics that deals with the interconversions of energy forms
33 Negatively charged ions
35 Hydrogen-accepting coenzyme containing niacin

DIGESTION AND ABSORPTION OF FOOD NUTRIENTS

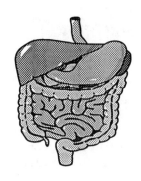

DEFINE KEY TERMS AND CONCEPTS

1. Hormone

2. Gastrointestinal tract

3. Alimentary canal

4. Mesentery

5. Hepatic-portal vein

6. Esophagus

7. Peristalsis

8. Sphincter

9. Stomach

10. Hydrochloric acid

11. Chyme

12. Rectum

13. Small intestine

14. Villi

15. Microvilli

16. Lacteals

17. Brush border

18. Segmentation contractions

19. Large intestine

20. Bile

21. Liver

22. Gall bladder

23. Pancreas

24. Emulsify

25. Colon

26. Ulcers

27. Autoregulatory control

28. Antacids

STUDY QUESTIONS

The gastrointestinal tract

List eight major structures of the GI tract.

1.   2.

3.   4.

5.   6.

7.   8.

What is the function of the mesentery and hepatic portal vein?

<u>Mesentery</u>

<u>Hepatic-portal vein</u>

Mouth and esophagus

Describe the role of the following structures in the digestive process:

Mouth

Pharynx

Esophagus

Esophageal sphincter

Describe the role of peristalsis in the digestive process.

What is a sphincter and what factors influence the activity of this structure during digestion?

Stomach

The parietal and chief cells of the gastric glands secrete two enzymes; identify and describe their functions.

	Enzyme	Function
Parietal cells		
Chief cells		

Small intestine

Identify and give the primary function of each of the three sections of the small intestine.

	Structure	Function
1.		
2.		
3.		

How do segmentation contractions differ from the contractions of peristalsis?

What happens when a lipid nutrient is emulsified?

Large intestine

List the six major components of the large intestine.

1.   4.

2.   5.

3.   6.

PRACTICE QUIZ
MULTIPLE CHOICE

1. Hormones are:
    a. protein-like substances
    b. deactivated in the stomach
    c. carbohydrate-like substances
    d. primarily produced in fat cells
    e. all of the above

2. The stomach secretes:
    a. hydrochloric acid
    b. pepsinogen
    c. carbonic acid
    d. mucous
    e. a, b, d
    f. all of the above

3. Digestion in the small intestine occurs primarily in:
    a. the duodenum
    b. the jejunum
    c. the ileum
    d. the pylorus

4. The large intestine consists of the:
    a. ascending colon and sigmoid colon
    b. villi
    c. transverse colon
    d. a and c
    e. all of the above

5. Ulcers occur when:
    a. an excessive amount of HCl is secreted in the intestinal tract
    b. gastric juices are not neutralized before they reach the intestinal lining
    c. a rough food particle tears the intestinal lining
    d. pepsinogen is secreted in excess into the intestine
    e. none of the above

FILL-IN

1. The _____ delivers nutrient-rich blood from the mesentery to the liver.

2. Food enters the stomach as the _____ relaxes.

3. The highly vascularized finger-like projections in the small intestine are called _____ .

4. Lyphatic vessels called _____ transport fatty materials from the digestive tract into the lymphatic vessels that eventually drain into the large vessels near the heart.

5. _____ is secreted from the gallbladder to aid in the emulsification of lipids.

TRUE / FALSE

____ 1. The absorption of nutrients takes place mainly in the stomach.

____ 2. Chyme is a slushy, non-acidic mixture of ingested food and secretions from the stomach lining.

____ 3. The absorptive surface of the small intestine, if spread out, would be the size of a tennis court.

____ 4. Bacteria aid in digestion by fermenting the remaining food residue in the large intestine.

____ 5. The main secretions of the large intestine are mucus and bicarbonates.

ACROSS

1 Made up of esophagus, gallbladder, liver, stomach, pancreas, intestines, rectum, and anus
7 Connective tissue that supports intestinal organs
9 Food passes from the esophagus into this organ
10 Finger-like protrusions of the intestinal mucosa
11 Bile is produced in this organ
15 Smooth muscle contractions that mix and move food along
17 Small projections on the villi through which nutrients are absorbed
21 The pyloric sphincter serves as the gateway into this intestine
22 Another term for the large intestine
23 Food passes through the phyarynx and enters this portion of the GI tract
24 Peristalsis involves progressive and recurring waves of smooth muscle _____

Chapter 2

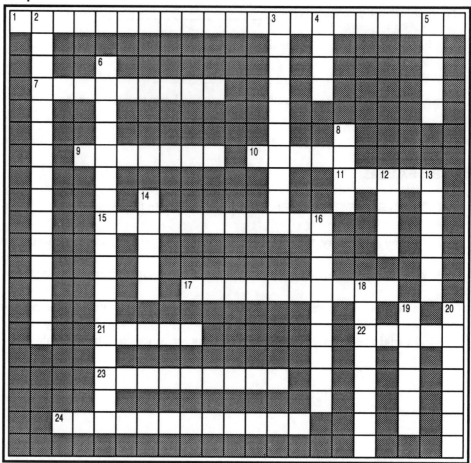

DOWN

2 Also called GI tract
3 Small and large _____
4 pH of the gastric juices in the stomach
5 Slushy, acidic mixture of food and digestive juices
6 Delivers nutrient-rich blood from intestine to liver
8 Gallbladder secretion that emulsifies fats
12 Hepatic-portal _____
13 Remnants of digestion are eliminated through this GI structure
14 _____ border

16 Smooth muscle ring that regulates food movement in the GI tract
18 Small lymphatic vessels within intestinal villi
19 Painful intestinal disorder
20 Also called GI tract

3 CARBOHYDRATES

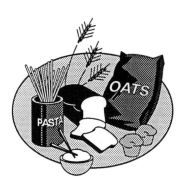

DEFINE KEY TERMS AND CONCEPTS

1. Carbohydrates

2. Pentoses

3. Hexoses

4. Monosaccharides

5. Glucose

6. Fructose

7. Galactose

8. Disaccharide

9. Sucrose

10. Maltose

11. Lactose

12. Simple sugars

13. Calorie

14. Polysaccharide

15. Starch

16. Cellulose

17. Bran layer

18. Dietary fiber

19. Water-soluble fibers

20. Water-insoluble fibers

21. Recommended fiber intake

22. Glycogen

23. Glycogenesis

24. Glycogenolysis

25. Cortisol

26. Gluconeogenesis

27. Insulin

28. Glucagon

29. Normoglycemic

30. Ketones

31. Hypoglycemia

32. Hyperglycemia

33. Diabetes mellitus

34. Salivary glands

35. Pancreatic amylase

36. Maltase

37. Sucrase

38. Lactase

39. Lactose intolerance

40. Hepatic-portal circulation

41. Feces

42. Hemorrhoids

STUDY QUESTIONS

What are carbohydrates?

How does the number of carbon atoms vary among carbohydrates?

Monosaccharides

List the three most common hexose monosaccharides in the diet and give a food source for each.

Monosaccharide	Food source
1. _____	_____
2. _____	_____
3. _____	_____

Disaccharides

How are disaccharides formed in nature?

Give the makeup of the following three common dietary disaccharides.

1. Sucrose = _____ + _____

2. Maltose = _____ + _____

3. Lactose = _____ + _____

How much simple sugar is consumed in the typical American diet?

Polysaccharides

What is a polysaccharide?

Identify three common forms of polysaccharide.

1.

2.

3.

What is starch?

What is dietary fiber?

List five kinds of dietary fiber.

1.   4.

2.   5.

3.

Discuss the possible beneficial role of dietary fiber on gastrointestinal function and blood cholesterol.

Gastrointestinal function

Blood cholesterol

What are some potential negative effects of an excessive intake of dietary fiber?

Indicate the average quantity of glycogen stored in:

Liver

Muscle

What role do the following hormones play in the regulation of blood glucose?

Insulin

Cortisol

Glucagon

Where do carbohydrates come from?

Outline the formation of carbohydrate in the process of photosynthesis.

Functions of carbohydrate

List and discuss the four major functions of carbohydrate in the body.

1.

2.

3.

4.

Recommended intake of carbohydrates

What is the recommended carbohydrate intake for physically active men and women?

Give two examples of how diet can affect the body's carbohydrate reserves.

1.

2.

Carbohydrates in foods

List five foods that are rich sources of carbohydrate.

1.   4.

2.   5.

3.

Digestion and absorption

Outline the process of carbohydrate digestion and absorption in the body.

Indicate the major digestive enzymes of carbohydrates and their specific action.

	Enzyme	Action
1.		
2.		
3.		

What is the major role of the hepatic-portal circulation in the absorption of food nutrients?

PRACTICE QUIZ

MULTIPLE CHOICE

1. Carbohydrates:
   a. are water-soluble organic compounds
   b. are made up of atoms of C, O, N, and H
   c. are made up of atoms of C, N, and O
   d. contain H and O atoms in the ratio of 1 to 1
   e. c and d

2. The most common forms of simple carbohydrate in the diet:
   a. are called pentoses
   b. contain 5 carbon atoms
   c. contain 6 carbon atoms
   d. are called hexoses
   e. c and d

3. In the body, glucose can be:
   a. used directly by the cell for energy
   b. stored as glycogen in the muscles and liver
   c. converted to fat for energy storage
   d. b and c
   e. all of the above

4. The disaccharide sucrose is formed from the union of the monosaccharides:
   a. glucose and glucose
   b. fructose and galactose
   c. fructose and fructose
   d. glucose and fructose

5. Which of the following statements are TRUE concerning polysaccharides?
   a. The term polysaccharide is used when two or more simple sugar molecules combine
   b. The most common polysaccharides are starch, fiber, and sucrose
   c. Most carbohydrates in plants are in the form of polysaccharides
   d. In the small intestine, polysaccharides are readily absorbed directly into the blood

FILL-IN

1. The major monosaccharides in the diet are _____ , _____ , and _____ .

2. The disaccharide _____ is the chief sugar present in milk.

3. _____ fiber is the classification for the type of dietary fiber that has been shown to have a lowering effect on blood cholesterol.

4. The process of synthesizing glucose from the structural components of other nutrients is termed _____ .

5. The hormone _____ , termed the insulin "antagonist," is secreted by the alpha cells of the pancreas.

TRUE / FALSE

_____ 1. Glucose is an example of a hexose sugar containing five carbon atoms in its molecular structure.

_____ 2. The sweetest of the monosaccharides is galactose.

_____ 3. The average American consumes about 50% of dietary carbohydrate as simple sugar in the predominant form of sucrose and high-fructose corn syrup.

_____ 4. The monosaccharides and polysaccharides collectively are called starch.

_____ 5. A rapid and large influx of glucose into the bloodstream can trigger a hormonal response that actually causes the blood sugar level to drop.

Chapter 3

ACROSS

2 Exposed rectal blood vessels that can be very painful

4 Six-carbon sugars

5 Glucose + galactose produces this sugar

6 Steroid hormone from the adrenal cortex

7 Enzyme required for lactose breakdown

10 Hormone secreted in hypoglycemia

12 Name for a basic sugar

13 Enzyme that facilitates maltose breakdown

17 Byproducts of incomplete fat breakdown

19 Hormone secreted in hyperglycemia

21 Fibrous covering of whole grains

22 Name of plant polysaccharide

DOWN

1 Semi-solid waste product expelled from the rectum

3 _____ - portal vein

4 Name for low blood sugar

8 Pancreatic hormone for starch breakdown

9 Enzyme that splits disaccharide to glucose + fructose

11 Disease of inadequate insulin production

12 Glucose + fructose

14 Water fibers do not lower cholesterol

15 Fibrous material in protective outer layer of whole grains

16 Complex carbohydrates in their natural state

18 Water fibers that do lower cholesterol

20 Typical American diet contains about 12g of this; may help prevent some forms of cancer

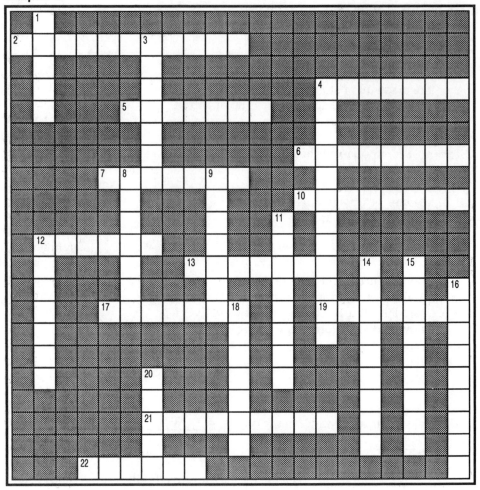

4 LIPIDS

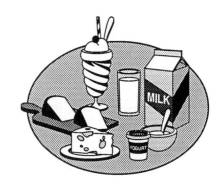

1. Lipid

2. Fats

3. Oils

4. Glycerol

5. Triglyceride

6. Compound fats

7. Derived fats

8. Fatty acids

9. Short-chain fatty acids

10. Medium-chain fatty acids

11. Long-chain fatty acids

12. Saturated fatty acids

13. Unsaturated fatty acids

14. Monounsaturated

15. Polyunsaturated

16. Omega-3 family of fatty acids

17. Phospholipids

18. Lecithin

19. Glycolipids

20. Cholesterol

21. Exogenous cholesterol

22. Endogenous cholesterol

23. Lipoproteins

24. Apoprotein

25. Chylomicron

26. Lipoprotein lipase

27. VLDL

28. HDL

29. LDL

30. IDL

31. Plaque

32. Essential fat

33. Anorexia nervosa

34. P/S ratio

35. Hydrogenation

36. Trans-fatty acid

37. Lingual lipase

38. Gastric lipase

39. Bile

40. Pancreatic lipase

41. Cholecystokinin

42. Gastric inhibitory peptide

43. Secretin

STUDY QUESTIONS

What are lipids?

   Composition of lipids

      Describe the molecular composition of the most common form of lipid in the body.

   Fatty acids

      What is meant by the terms "saturated" and "unsaturated" fatty acid? Give two examples of each.

         <u>Saturated</u>

            <u>Example 1</u>

<u>Example 2</u>

<u>Unsaturated</u>

<u>Example 1</u>

<u>Example 2</u>

Saturated fat intake

What is the P/S ratio recommended for health reasons?

Indicate the typical amount of saturated fat intake for Americans. Excess intake of saturated fat can cause what disease?

<u>Saturated fat intake</u>

<u>Disease</u>

Ratio of polyunsaturated to saturated fats

What is a desirable ratio of saturated-to-polyunsaturated fat in the diet?

Ratio of saturated-to-monounsaturated-to-polyunsaturated fatty acids

What is the recommended ratio of saturated-to-monounsaturated-to-polyunsaturated fat in the diet?

High fat diets and cancer

What is the association between a diet high in fat and the incidence of cancer?

Phospholipids and related fats

List one phospholipid and its major function in the body.

<u>Phospholipid</u>   <u>Function</u>

Cholesterol

What is the major dietary source of cholesterol? What are some important functions of cholesterol in the body?

<u>Dietary source</u>

<u>Functions</u>

Cholesterol and heart disease risk

What effect does reducing blood cholesterol have on heart disease risk?

All of the data are not in

List two controversies regarding cholesterol and heart disease.

1.

2.

The lipoproteins: fat carriers in the bloodstream

How are lipids transported in the bloodstream?

High -and low-density lipoproteins

What are two main types of lipoproteins and their function?

	Type	Function
1.		
2.		

Bad cholesterol /good cholesterol

Identify "bad" and "good" cholesterol and their main function in the body.

	Proper name	Function
"Bad" cholesterol		
"Good" cholesterol		

Unsaturated and saturated fats

List three major differences between unsaturated and saturated fat.

1.

2.

3.

Fat intake

List three major sources of dietary fat intake in the American diet.

1.

2.

3.

Margarine versus butter

Describe two differences between butter and margarine.

1.

2.

A health risk in trans-fatty acids

How are trans-fatty acids formed in the production of margarine?

Fish oils may be healthful

What food sources contain omega-3 fatty acids, and how are these fatty acids related to heart disease risk?

Sources

Relation to CHD

Functions of lipids

List the six major functions of lipids in the body.

1.   4.

2.   5.

3.   6.

Energy source

An energy-rich fuel

What aspect of the chemical structure of fat causes it to contain more energy than an equal weight of carbohydrate?

Protection of vital organs

Insulation

Discuss the role of body fat as an insulator and protector of vital organs.

Other functions

Vitamin carrier

List the four vitamins stored in body fat.

1.

2.

3.

4.

Satiety

Why do many reducing diets contain some fat?

Biological membranes

How do lipids control the passage of substances into and out of cells?

Essential nutrients

List two essential polyunsaturated fatty acids.

1.

2.

Fat content of common foods

In the typical American diet, what percent of lipid is derived from vegetable and animal origin?

<u>Vegetable origin</u>

<u>Animal origin</u>

Digestion and absorption

Outline the process of digestion and absorption of dietary fat.

PRACTICE QUIZ

MULTIPLE CHOICE

1. A lipid:
   a. has the molecular formula $C_6H_{12}O_6$
   b. can have fatty acid chains of different lengths
   c. can be of plant or animal origin
   d. b and c
   e. all of the above

2. Saturated fats are found in:
   a. chocolate
   b. corn oil
   c. sunflower seeds
   d. cold-water fish
   e. all of the above

3. The recommended P/S ratios:
   a. 0.5/1
   b. 0.75/1
   c. 0.5/1
   d. 4/1
   e. 1/1

4. Phospholipids:
   a. have a unit containing a phosphate instead of a fatty acid chain
   b. are a crucial element of the plasma membrane
   c. are important in blood clotting
   d. are part of the myelin sheath around nerve fibers
   e. all of the above

5. Cholesterol is important because:
   a. it is a component in the synthesis of bile
   b. it aids in the production of estrogen, androgen, and progesterone
   c. it aids in liver function
   d. it is a part of cell membranes
   e. a, b, and d

FILL-IN

1. Fatty acids with at least one double bond are called _____.

2. The most abundant type of fat in the human body is in the form of _____.

3. If a fatty acid chain contains two or more double bonds it is said to be _____.

4. One gram of fat contains approximately _____ calories.

5. Recommended daily fat intake should be below _____ percent of total intake.

TRUE / FALSE

_____ 1. On a per weight basis, carbohydrates contain more energy than lipids.

_____ 2. Glycerol combines with three fatty acid chains to form a triglyceride molecule.

_____ 3. Saturated fats are present only in animal tissues.

_____ 4. Cholesterol is a fat-like substance that contains more calories per gram than unsaturated fat.

_____ 5. One gram of dietary fat contains more potential energy than either protein or carbohydrate.

Chapter 4

ACROSS

2 Lipids in solid form at room temperature
7 Fatty acids with 8 to 12 carbon atoms
9 No double bonds in carbon chain
11 Enzyme that facilitates hydrolysis of triglycerides
12 Anorexia _____
14 Cholesterol synthesized by the body
17 Abbreviation for lipoprotein formed when VLDL is acted upon by lipoprotein lipase
19 Abbreviation for lipoprotein containing largest percentage of lipid
20 Cholesterol obtained in the diet
22 Phospholipid compound that helps regulate the passage of lipids through the cell membrane
23 Fatty acids in corn oil

DOWN

1 Non-fat component of triglyceride molecule
3 By far, the most plentiful form of fat in the body
4 Lipids in liquid form
5 Ratio of polyunsaturated to saturated fats in the diet
6 Margarine has 17 to 25% of these total fatty acids, butter only 7%
8 Abbreviation for "good" cholesterol
10 Fatty acids with 4 to 8 carbon atoms
13 Triglyceride = glycerol plus 3 fatty _____
15 Form of fatty acid found in fish oils

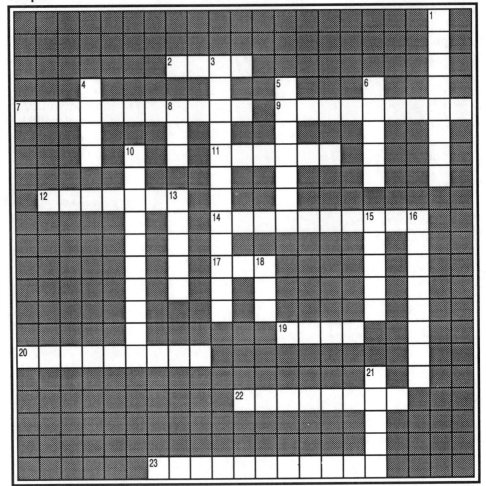

16 Hormone released when there is a high fat content in the stomach to reduce gastric motility
18 Abbreviation for "bad" cholesterol
21 Another name for fat

5 PROTEINS

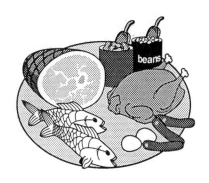

1. Proteins

2. Amino acids

3. Peptide bonds

4. Dipeptide

5. Tripeptide

6. Polypeptide

7. Structural proteins

8. Hemoglobin

9. Sickle-cell anemia

10. Essential

11. Nonessential

12. Transamination

13. Deamination

14. Osteoblasts

15. Myofilaments

16. Hemoglobin

17. Hormones

18. Endocrine glands

19. Recommended Dietary Allowance

20. U.S. RDA

21. ESADDI

22. U.S. RDA for protein

23. Positive nitrogen balance

24. Negative nitrogen balance

25. High quality protein

26. Lower quality protein

27. Index of Nutritional Quality

28. Biologic value

29. Vegans

30. Lacto-vegetarian

31. Lacto-ovovegetarian

32. Gastrin

33. Trypsin

34. Trypsinogen

What are proteins?

How does the chemical structure of proteins differ from lipids and carbohydrates?

Amino acids

Draw the basic chemical structure of an amino acid molecule. (Hint: refer to Figure 5-1 in the texbook.)

What is transamination, and of what advantage is this process to the body's amino acid needs?

What is the chemical distinction between a dipeptide, tripeptide, and polypeptide?

Dipeptide

Tripeptide

Polypeptide

What is the cause and what is the effect of sickle cell anemia?

Cause

Effect

Essential and nonessential amino acids

What is the primary difference between essential and nonessential amino acids?

Where do proteins come from?
  Dietary sources

List common dietary sources of animal and plant protein.

<u>Animal protein</u>

<u>Plant protein</u>

Synthesis in the body

How are nonessential amino acids synthesized in the body?

Give one example of the process of transamination and one of deamination.

<u>Transamination</u>

<u>Deamination</u>

Functions of protein

What is meant by the "anabolic" role of protein in body processes?

Structural components of body tissues

List 10 body structures, tissues, or compounds of which protein is an important component.

1.   6.

2.   7.

3.   8.

4.   9.

5.   10.

Other functions of proteins

List two plasma proteins and their primary function.

<u>Plasma protein</u>   <u>Primary function</u>

1.

2.

The Recommended Dietary Allowance

What is the RDA?

Why is it important for a person to regularly consume the RDA for a particular nutrient?

The United States Recommended Daily Allowance

What is the U.S. RDA?

What is the adult U.S. RDA for protein for a woman who weighs 122 lb and for a man who weighs 176 lb?
(Hint: convert lb to kg.)

<u>Protein RDA for the woman</u>

<u>Protein RDA for the man</u>

What does it mean when the body is said to be in protein balance?

What can happen to lean body mass during weight loss on a very low calorie diet?

Proteins in food

List specific high quality and lower quality dietary proteins.

High quality protein

Lower quality protein

List the four major sources of protein in the American diet.

1.   3.

2.   4.

Nutrient density

What is meant by the term "nutrient density"?

List the five steps to compute the INQ for protein in one raw egg.

Step 1.

Step 2.

Step 3.

Step 4.

Step 5.

Vegetarian approach to sound nutrition

Indicate three particular nutritional problem areas for men and women on a vegetarian diet.

1.

2.

3.

What are the differences between a strict vegan diet, a lacto-vegetarian diet, and an lacto-ovovegetarian diet?

Vegan diet

Lacto-vegetarian diet

Lacto-ovovegetarian diet

Digestion and absorption

Give the function of the stomach enzymes pepsin and gastrin in protein digestion.

Pepsin

Gastrin

Indicate three events that can occur when amino acids reach the liver.

1.

2.

3.

MULTIPLE CHOICE

1. Protein:
   a. provides between 15-25% of the body's energy
   b. can be a source for synthesizing glucose
   c. has the same dietary requirement for growing children as for adults
   d. if taken in amounts above the RDA will induce muscular growth during strength training
   e. b and d

2. The RDA represents:
   a. the minimum nutrient requirement for health
   b. a liberal estimate of the quantity of a particular nutrient required to sustain good health
   c. a liberal yet safe estimate of nutritional needs
   d. a and b
   e. b and c

3. High protein diets:
   a. place an extra strain on the liver and kidneys
   b. generally cause a temporary increase in the metabolic rate due to a large SDA effect
   c. increase the requirement for water intake
   d. a and c
   e. all of the above

4. Which of the following statements are TRUE?
   a. The healthy adult human requires eight essential amino acids
   b. A complete protein contains all of the essential amino acids in the proportions required for bodily function and growth
   c. Eggs, meat, milk, and cheese are considered high quality proteins
   d. An incomplete protein is a food source that contains a low quantity of protein
   e. a, b, and c

5. When protein is used for energy:
   a. it first must be deaminated in the liver
   b. a portion of the potential energy in the amino acid molecule is lost to the body via the hydrogen excreted as NH_2
   c. it can add to the body's water loss and may create a state of dehydration
   d. all of the above

FILL-IN

1. In terms of overall size, a protein molecule usually contains a minimum of _____ amino acids.

2. Amino acids are joined by _____.

3. When an amino group is removed from an amino acid molecule, the process is called _____.

4. The nutritional quality of a particular food can be evaluated by determining its _____.

5. A _____ diet allows the addition of milk and related products such as cheese.

TRUE / FALSE

_____ 1. Regular exercise causes an increase in the requirement for dietary protein above the RDA.

_____ 2. The athlete in heavy training generally has greater difficulty obtaining adequate caloric intake on a vegetarian diet compared to a non-vegetarian counterpart.

_____ 3. Vegetarian diets are generally high in fiber, vitamins, and minerals.

_____ 4. The protein in nervous and connective tissue is essentially fixed, whereas muscle protein can be altered and used for energy.

_____ 5. Compared to non-vegetarians, vegans generally have greater difficulty obtaining adequate quantities of calcium and phosphorous in non-fortified food sources.

Chapter 5

ACROSS

1 Process of forming amino acids within the body
4 Form of chemical bonding by which amino acids are linked
6 Nitrogen balance where intake exceeds excretion
9 Diet allows addition of milk and related products
12 All food intake is from plant kingdom
16 Nitrogen-containing macronutrients
19 Many amino acids linked together
20 Protein formed from two amino acids
21 0.8g/kg of body mass for protein intake

DOWN

1 Pancreatic enzyme; trypsin is inactive precursor
2 Nitrogen balance where excretion exceeds intake
3 Contractile elements within muscle fibers
5 Eight amino acids that must be consumed in the diet
7 Iron-protein compound within red blood cell
8 Three amino acids linked together
10 Bone-forming cells
11 Secret hormones directly into extracellular spaces
13 Building blocks of protein
14 Anemia caused by deformed red blood cells
15 Chemical messengers
17 _____ of nutritional quality
18 Quality of protein that contains all essential amino acids

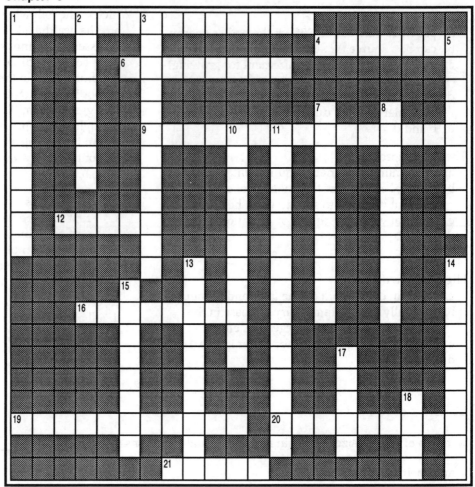

6 VITAMINS

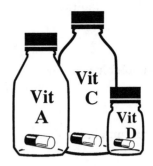

DEFINE KEY TERMS AND CONCEPTS

1. Vitamins

2. Coenzyme

3. Provitamin

4. Preformed vitamin

5. Scurvy

6. James Lind

7. Ascorbic acid

8. Casimir Funk

9. Vitamine

10. Vitamin supplements are big business

11. Fat-soluble vitamins

12. Water-soluble vitamins

13. Toxic accumulations

14. Retinol equivalent

15. Hypervitaminosis A

16. Excessive intake of vitamin D

17. Hypercalcemia

18. Synthesis of vitamins

19. Megavitamins

20. Vitamin C megadose

21. B-complex vitamins

22. Niacin excess

23. Pyridoxine supplementation

24. Excessive folic acid intake

25. Vitamin B$_{12}$

What are vitamins?

What is a vitamin?

In what way is a vitamin considered to be a chemical catalyst in the body?

The discovery of vitamins

Give a brief historical perspective on the discovery of vitamin C.

Classification of vitamins

Fat-soluble vitamins

List the fat-soluble vitamins and indicate their major functions in the body.

Vitamin	Function
1.	
2.	
3.	
4.	

Water-soluble vitamins

List the water-soluble vitamins and indicate their major functions in the body.

	Vitamin	Function
1.		
2.		
3.		
4.		
5.		
6.		
7.		
8.		
9.		

Recommended intake of vitamins

Indicate the vitamin RDAs for the American adult male and female.

Vitamin	Male	Female
A		
D		
E		
K		
C		
B_1		
B_2		
Niacin		
B_6		
Pantothenic acid		
Folic acid		
Biotin		
B_{12}		

Functions of vitamins

Indicate a major food source and function(s) for each of the fat- and water-soluble vitamins.

	Vitamin	Food source	Function
1.			
2.			
3.			
4.			
5.			
6.			
7.			
8.			
9.			
10.			
11.			
12.			
13.			

What is the primary role of water-soluble vitamins in human energy metabolism?

Vitamins and exercise performance

What is a primary reason many coaches and athletes believe that vitamin intake above the RDA is important to an athlete's diet?

A competitive edge

Discuss, using research findings, whether supplements above the RDA of the following vitamins enhance exercise performance.

Vitamin B_6

Vitamin C

Vitamin E

Toxicity of fat-soluble vitamins

Give an example of how a megadose of fat-soluble vitamins can pose a danger to good health.

Digestion and absorption

Indicate the sites for the absorption of the various fat- and water-soluble vitamins.

PRACTICE QUIZ

MULTIPLE CHOICE

1. The amine substance isolated from rice polishings that cured the disease beriberi was first identified by:
   a. Vasco de Gama
   b. James Lind
   c. Sir Frederick Hopkins
   d. Casimir Funk

2. Which vitamin promotes growth and mineralization of bones and increases absorption of calcium:
   a. vitamin A
   b. vitamin D
   c. vitamin C
   d. vitamin K

3. Vitamins ____ and ____ pose the greatest risk to good health if regularly consumed in excess because they can accumulate to reach toxic levels:
   a. E and D
   b. D and A
   c. A and the B-complex
   d. C and E
   e. none of the above

4. The water-soluble vitamins are different from their fat-soluble counterparts in that:
   a. they must be consumed regularly--usually daily or within a several-day period
   b. they can routinely be consumed in excess above the RDA without any health risk
   c. they are inorganic compounds
   d. they are composed of vitamin C and four vitamins from the B-complex group
   e. a and c

5. A potential significant positive effect of vitamins C, A, and E is to:
   a. serve as a protective antioxidant and reducing agent to blunt potential cellular damage from free radical attack
   b. reduce the frequency and duration of the common cold
   c. facilitate energy metabolism, thus enhancing exercise performance
   d. all of the above

FILL-IN

1. The chemical name for the vitamin that protects against scurvy is _____ .

2. About _____ % of Americans regularly supplement with vitamins.

3. A megadose of vitamins is an intake that exceeds the RDA by at least _____ -fold.

4. _____ different vitamins have been isolated, analyzed, and synthesized and their RDA levels established.

5. _____ is the only vitamin that is not available in a strict vegetarian diet.

TRUE / FALSE

_____ 1. A retinol equivalent or RE is a measure of vitamin D activity.

_____ 2. Vitamin supplementation above the RDA level is not related to improved exercise performance .

_____ 3. The capacity for vitamin synthesis in the animal kingdom far exceeds that observed for plants.

_____ 4. Vitamins obtained preformed naturally in food are rated as higher quality than vitamins commercially synthesized in the laboratory.

_____ 5. Essentially there is no difference in the vitamin content of fresh fruits and vegetables and the same vegetables that are canned or frozen.

Chapter 6

ACROSS

3 Form of Vitamin A
5 Some vitamins are soluble in _____
7 An inactive precursor form of vitamin
8 Essential organic substances that perform specific metabolic functions
9 Chemical name of vitamin C
14 An active vitamin from food or supplements
18 Combining separate elements to create new ones
19 Some vitamins are water soluble; others are

_____ _____

DOWN

1 This vitamin may be beneficial during pregnancy
2 Polish chemist
4 Megadose of vitamin A can be _____
6 Unites with a protein compound to form an active enzyme
10 Citrus fruits cured this disease on sailing ships in the 1700s
11 Vitamins sold in this form are big business
12 More than 10 times the RDA
13 Physician researcher who tried to cure scurvy
15 Casimir Funk discovered these vital substances
16 Can cause flushing or redness of skin if taken in excess
17 RDA is 60 mg for this vitamin that is plentiful in citrus fruits.

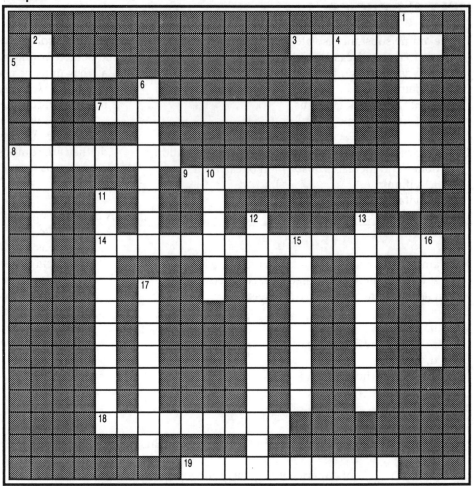

7 MINERALS

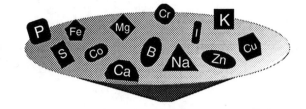

DEFINE KEY TERMS AND CONCEPTS

1. Minerals

2. Major minerals

3. Trace minerals

4. Bioavailability

5. Vitamin-mineral interaction

6. Fiber-mineral interactions

7. Phytate

8. Oxalate

9. Iodine

10. Thyroxine

11. Iodized salt

12. Iron insufficiency

13. Calcium

14. Hydroxyapatite

15. Osteoporosis

16. Estrogen

17. Menopause

18. Secondary amenorrhea

19. Phosphorus

20. Magnesium

21. Sodium

22. Potassium

23. Chlorine

24. Electrolytes

25. Aldosterone

26. Sodium-induced hypertension

27. Iron

28. Hemoglobin

29. Myoglobin

30. Cytochromes

31. Iron deficiency anemia

32. Sports anemia

33. Clinical anemia

34. Heat cramps

35. Heat exhaustion

36. Heat stroke

STUDY QUESTIONS

What are minerals?

What is the difference between a major mineral and a trace mineral?

<u>Major mineral</u>

<u>Trace mineral</u>

Bioavailability

What two factors influence the bioavailability of minerals?

1.

2.

Where do minerals come from?

Identify two sources of minerals in the diet.

1.

2.

Functions of minerals

List three major functions of minerals in the body.

1.

2.

3.

Recommended intake and source of minerals

    Minerals in food: their relation to physical activity

      Calcium

List five functions of calcium in the body.

1.

2.

3.

4.

5.

Osteoporosis: calcium, estrogen, and exercise

What happens to the bones when calcium intake is deficient?

A progressive disease

Outline the typical progression of osteoporosis.

Dietary calcium is crucial

Identify two major dietary sources of calcium.

1.

2.

Exercise is helpful

What is the proposed role of exercise as a "treatment" for osteoporosis?

Is too much training harmful?

Under what conditions can too much exercise be harmful to the bone mass, particularly for females?

Phosphorus

Why is phosphorous considered a versatile mineral in body functions?

Magnesium

List four functions of magnesium in the body.

1.

2.

3.

4.

Sodium, potassium, and chlorine

Indicate the function of the following electrolytes in the body.

<u>Electrolyte</u>   <u>Function</u>

Sodium

Potassium

Chlorine

Sodium: how much is enough?

What is the recommended dietary intake of sodium, and the possible result of a chronic excess sodium intake?

<u>Recommended sodium intake</u>

<u>Effect of sodium excess</u>

Iron

What is the body's normal iron content for males and females?

<u>Males</u>

<u>Females</u>

Primarily related to energy metabolism

Describe three important functions of iron in the body other than its role in oxygen transport.

1.

2.

3.

Iron stores

Identify potential consequences of a prolonged iron-deficient diet.

The source of iron is important

List two sources of dietary iron.

1.

2.

Females: a population at risk

Who are more likely, men or women, to exhibit a significant iron insufficiency? Discuss.

Exercise-induced anemia: fact or fiction?

Discuss three factors that could contribute to the occurrence of "sports anemia."

1.

2.

3.

Minerals and exercise performance

What are the effects of long-duration exercise on mineral loss, especially in hot weather?

Digestion and absorption

"Both intrinsic and extrinsic factors control the eventual fate of ingested minerals." Discuss.

PRACTICE QUIZ

MULTIPLE CHOICE

1. Minerals are found in:
   a. enzymes
   b. hormones
   c. vitamins
   d. intracellular fluids
   e. all of the above

2. Which of the following are trace minerals:
   a. potassium
   b. zinc
   c. sodium
   d. calcium
   e. none of the above

3. Which of the following foods can help achieve appropriate iron intake in iron-deficient individuals:
   a. peaches
   b. leafy green vegetables
   c. non-fat yogurt
   d. cheese
   e. b, c, and d
   f. all of the above

4. Some of the major roles minerals play in body function include:
   a. regulate cellular metabolism
   b. provide structure for bones and teeth
   c. function to maintain normal heart rhythm, muscle contractility, and nerve conduction
   d. regulate hormonal control of secondary sex characteristics
   e. all of the above

5. Calcium plays an important role in:
   a. muscle contraction
   b. blood clotting
   c. thyroid activity
   d. heart contraction
   e. a, b, and d
   f. all of the above

FILL-IN

1. A major dietary source of calcium is _____ .

2. Nerve transmission is one of the major body functions in which the group of minerals called _____ is involved.

3. If a person is deficient in iodine, he/she may suffer from _____ .

4. _____ is the compound synthesized from calcium and phosphorous to form teeth and bones.

5. _____ is the condition where bones lose their mineral mass and progressively become porous and brittle.

TRUE / FALSE

_____ 1. Consuming greater than 35 grams of dietary fiber daily can decrease the absorption of certain minerals.

_____ 2. It is essential that some minerals such as zinc, magnesium, and iron be supplemented because they cannot be obtained adequately in a well-balanced diet.

_____ 3. All the minerals humans need can be obtained from a well-balanced diet.

_____ 4. Exercise generally provides a stimulus to maintain and even increase bone mass in adults.

_____ 5. Phosphorous plays a key role in the structure of DNA and RNA.

Chapter 7

ACROSS

3 An organic compound found in grain fibers and coffee

4 Absorption of this mineral is facilitated by vitamin C intake

7 Common name for sodium chloride

8 These minerals are required in amounts less than 100 mg a day

11 Important mineral component of a hormone that accelerates resting metabolism

13 Iron-protein compound that stores and transports oxygen within muscle

15 This mineral is part of the compound that transforms energy for all biologic work

18 Complete cessation of menstruation

20 Important extracellular electrolyte

21 The body is composed of these 22 mostly metallic elements

23 Most abundant mineral in the body

24 Classification of anemia defined as hemoglobin levels of 12 g per 100 ml or less for women

25 A risk of untreated hypertension

26 Symptom of heat illness related to involuntary muscle spasms

DOWN

1 Consuming too much of this plant polysaccharide actually decreases absorption of certain minerals

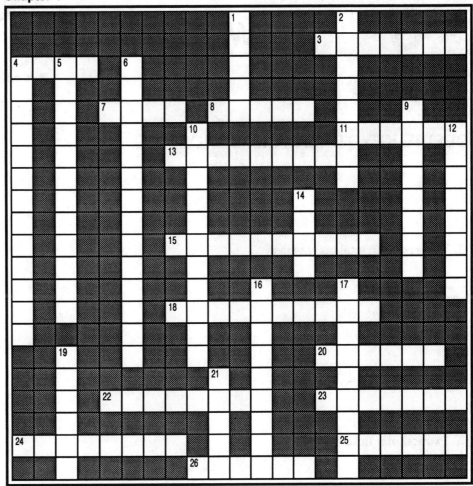

2 Mineral component of table salt

4 Anemia is an extreme condition of iron _____

5 Disease characterized by "brittle bones"

6 Heat disorder characterized by weak, rapid pulse, weakness, and ineffective circulatory adjustments

9 Essential substances needed by the body in minute amounts to perform highly specific metabolic functions

10 Depot of heme iron founds in specialized chains of these enzymes

12 Hormone often prescribed to treat side effects of menopause

14 Mineral required for the transfer of electrons during energy metabolism

16 Important intracellular electrolyte

17 Bone mass decreases greatly during this phase of a woman's life

19 Condition in which blood hemoglobin is significantly below normal

21 Those minerals required in amounts greater than 100 mg a day

8 WATER

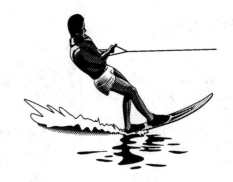

1. Water

2. Differences in total body water

3. Gender differences

4. Intracellular fluid (ICF)

5. Extracellular fluid (ECF)

6. Sources of water intake and output

7. Metabolic water

8. Urine

9. Insensible perspiration

10. Sweat

11. Dehydration

12. Evaporation

13. Intestinal elimination

14. Relative humidity

15. Factors that influence gastric emptying

16. Hyperthermia

17. Hyponatremia

18. Polymerized glucose

STUDY QUESTIONS

Water in the body

What are the gender differences in the body's water content, and what factors account for these differences?

<u>Males</u>

<u>Females</u>

Fluid compartments

What are the differences in location, amount, and chemical characteristics of intracellular and extracellular water?

<u>Intracellular water</u>

<u>Extracellular water</u>

Functions of body water

List three important functions of body water.

1.

2.

3.

Water balance: intake versus output

Water intake

List and quantify three primary sources of the daily intake of fluid.

<u>Source</u>   <u>Amount</u>

1.

2.

3.

Water output

List and quantify four primary sources of the daily water output.

<u>Source</u>   <u>Amount</u>

1.

2.

3.

4.

What is meant when we say: "Evaporation of sweat provides the refrigeration to cool the body?"

Water requirements in exercise

Practical recommendations for fluid replacement

Give three practical recommendations for fluid replacement when exercising in the heat.

1.

2.

3.

Gastric emptying

List three factors that influence the rate of gastric emptying of ingested fluids.

1.

2.

3.

Adequacy of rehydration

What is the danger of dehydration and how can it be prevented?

<u>Danger</u>

<u>Prevention</u>

Use of glucose polymers

What is the advantage of consuming sport drinks composed of glucose polymers versus drinks containing simple sugars?

PRACTICE QUIZ

MULTIPLE CHOICE

1. Of the four ways that water is lost from the body, which provides the greatest output:
   - a. feces
   - b. lungs
   - c. skin
   - d. urine

2. People who sweat heavily during exercise should:
   - a. take a salt tablet whenever a cramp occurs
   - b. eat bananas because they are high in potassium
   - c. regularly replace the water lost through sweating
   - d. slowly become acclimatized so their sweat glands won't sweat as much
   - e. take a cold drink with concentrated sugar

3. The water needs of the body are supplied from these main sources:
   - a. liquids, fruits, vegetables
   - b. foods, fluids, metabolism
   - c. fruits, liquids, solids
   - d. lipids, proteins, carbohydrates
   - e. respiration, ATP breakdown, metabolism

4. Under normal conditions, a maximum of about 9.5 liters of water can be consumed daily without kidney strain or dilution of important chemicals. Consuming more than this volume may:
   - a. deaminate all excess proteins and convert them to dextromaltins
   - b. transform polymerized glucose into an unstable compound
   - c. produce hyponatremia (dilution of the body's normal sodium concentration)
   - d. cause large amounts of hydrogen and oxygen to combine
   - e. trigger a depressed urine output and subsequent dehydration

5. A carbohydrate-rich, vegetarian diet produces an alkaline urine, while high-protein diets:
   - a. produce an acidic urine with pH = 7.3 to 9.0
   - b. produce an acidic urine with a pH below 7.0
   - c. produce an alkaline urine with pH = 2.5 to 4.5
   - d. cause proteinuria, albuminuria, bilirubinuria, and ketonuria
   - e. cause excessive dehydration and alkalosis

FILL-IN

1. In the disease _____, urine has a fruit-like smell due to the presence of the chemical acetone.

2. A small quantity of water, perhaps 350 ml, continually seeps from the deeper tissues through the skin to the body's surface. This loss of water is called _____ perspiration.

3. In hot weather, much water is lost through the skin in the form of _____.

4. _____ refers to the water content of the air in relation to the total content it is capable of holding.

5. A dangerously elevated body temperature is called _____.

TRUE / FALSE

_____1. The energy content of a particular food is in general directly related to its water content.

_____2. The body water content of males ranges between 57 and 65% of body mass, while the water content of females ranges between 46 and 53%.

_____3. Solutions like blood, cytoplasm, and digestive juices are the media in which all biologic processes occur.

_____4. Normally, about 4.0 liters of water are required each day for a sedentary adult living under the normal range of environmental temperatures.

_____5. Fruits and vegetables (lettuce, pickles, green beans, broccoli) are generally low in water content, whereas the water contained in butter, chocolate, cookies, and cakes is quite high.

Chapter 8

ACROSS

1 Occurs when fluid loss is not matched by fluid replacement

4 Three _____ _____ _____ for the body are from liquids, foods, and metabolism

7 _____ emptying is slowed when the ingested fluid is concentrated with simple sugars

8 H_2O

9 This water is produced when the food macronutrients are degraded for energy

11 8 to 12 liters of this fluid can be produced during hot weather exercise

13 A dangerously elevated body temperature is called _____ thermia

17 Normally between 100 to 200 ml of water are lost through _____ elimination

DOWN

1 In adults, _____ ___ _____ body water among people are due to variations in body composition

2 Abbreviation referring to fluids within the cell

3 _____ _____ in total body water are due to differences in % body fat between men and women

5 Humidity expressed as the water content of air in relation to its total capacity to hold water

6 This process provides the refrigeration mechanism to cool the body

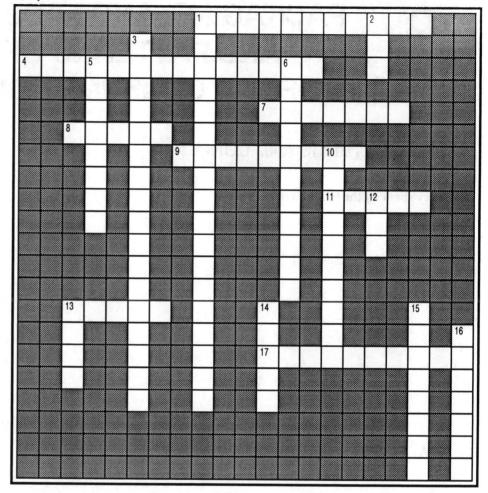

10 A form of perspiration occurring as water seeps from the deeper tissues through the skin

12 Abbreviation referring to all fluid outside of the cell

13 _____natremia is the clinical term for water intoxication

14 Normally, about 1.5 quarts of water are lost from the body in this form

15 Fluid in the joints

16 Polymerized sport drinks usually contain this form of simple sugar

9

FOOD ADVERTISING, PACKAGING, AND LABELING, AND PATTERNS OF FOOD CONSUMPTION

1. Money spent by the food industry

2. Governmental agencies

3. FTC

4. FDA

5. USDA

6. BATF

7. Organic

8. Natural

9. Sugar-free

10. Low calorie

11. Light

12. Imitation

13. Sodium-free

14. Low-sodium

15. Very low-sodium

16. Reduced-sodium

17. Fortified

18. Enriched

19. No cholesterol

20. Cholesterol-free

21. Low-fat

22. Fat-free

23. New

24. No artificial flavoring

25. No artificial coloring

26. Wheat

27. Fair Packaging and Labeling Act

28. U.S. RDA

29. Standard of identity

30. GRAS list

31. Pattern of food consumption

STUDY QUESTIONS

Food advertising

List three important factors that have stimulated the current interest in healthful patterns of eating.

1.

2.

3.

Advertising's goal is to shape behavior

Give two examples of how advertising impacts our behavior in terms of food consumption and exercise.

1.

2.

Governmental watchdog agencies

Identify and give the major function of the four agencies that oversee the food industry in the United States.

Agency   Function

1.

2.

3.

4.

Definitions used in advertising

Define 10 words or terms used in advertising that have a specific meaning in terms of federal regulations.

Term   Meaning

1.

2.

3.

4.

5.

6.

7.

8.

9.

10.

Food labeling

What is required by the Fair Packaging and Labeling Act?

By 1993, what specific additional information will be required to be placed on packages of processed food?

Food additives

List two purposes of the GRAS list.

    1.

    2.

Determining the percentage of a nutrient in a food

Choose a food that you ate for breakfast today (e.g., cereal) and list the specific macronutrients contained in this food and the percentage contribution of each to the total caloric content of the food.

Learn to read food labels

Choose a common food in your diet and evaluate its nutritional value based on the information appearing on the label. Include the percentage of carbohydrate, lipid, and protein in relation to the food's total caloric content.

Patterns of food consumption

Discuss two important factors that influence the quality and patterns of food consumption.

1.

2.

How much are we eating?

Outline the pattern of food consumption (macronutrients) in the U.S. over the last 20 years.

PRACTICE QUIZ

MULTIPLE CHOICE

1. In 1990, the food industry spent approximately how many dollars on food advertising and packaging:
   a. 400 million
   b. 10 billion
   c. 17 million
   d. 40 billion

2. The federal agency responsible for regulating media advertising of food products is:
   a. USDA
   b. FTC
   c. FCC
   d. FDA
   e. none of the above

3. Which of the following foods do not require federal inspection?
   a. fish
   b. meat
   c. poultry
   d. eggs
   e. a and d

4. A food label states: "This margarine will reduce your chances of heart disease." Which agency is responsible for evaluating the validity of this claim:
   a. FTC
   b. USDA
   c. FBI
   d. Bureau of Alcohol, Tobacco and Firearms
   e. none of the above

5. In food advertising, the term(s) _____ can be used if the product is sold as it occurs in nature and without additives, artificial flavoring, synthetic ingredients, preservatives, or coloring.
   a. enriched
   b. organic
   c. light
   d. natural
   e. a and d

FILL-IN

1. Approximately _____ percent of the meals eaten in the U.S. are now prepared outside of the home.

2. The term _____ can appear on a food label if vitamins and minerals have been added to the product if they were missing previously.

3. The _____ list provides a listing of food additives such as flavoring and coloring agents whose relative safety has been evaluated and established by the Food and Drug Administration.

4. When a modified food product contains one-third fewer calories or less than the regular product the term _____ can appear on the label and in advertising.

5. The federal regulatory agency responsible for the information contained on the labels for beer, wine, and liquor is the _____ .

TRUE / FALSE

_____ 1. A product is considered "fat-free" if it has less than one-half gram of fat per serving.

_____ 2. Recent data indicate that the quality of the food most commonly ordered by children and adolescents when eating out is quite similar to the nutritional guidelines of the American Heart Association.

_____ 3. Soft drink companies spend eight times more money to advertise than the dairy industry.

_____ 4. The FDA is directly responsible for regulating the food labelling of meat and poultry.

_____ 5. In 1988, each American spent approximately $1044 for food and alcoholic beverages consumed at home.

Chapter 9

ACROSS

5 Abbreviation for agency that regulates all food labeling except poultry and meat

6 List of food flavoring and coloring agents believed safe for human consumption

7 This word represents the final letter in the abbreviation of BATF

8 The Fair Packaging and _____ _____ was passed by Congress in 1966 to set standards for food labels

11 Term to describe a product as it occurs in nature without additives

13 Abbreviation for agency that regulates the labeling of meat and poultry

14 Product containing flavors only from naturally occurring products can be labeled "No artificial _____"

17 Term commonly used for products (e.g., beer) for which there are no regulations governing its use

19 Sodium content lowered by 75% compared to the original product can be labeled, "_____ sodium"

21 First word of the federal agency that decides what additives can be in food

22 Substituted product that resembles another food but is nutritionally inferior than the food it imitates

23 When applied to milk, this term indicates a fat content of between 0.5 and 2.0 percent

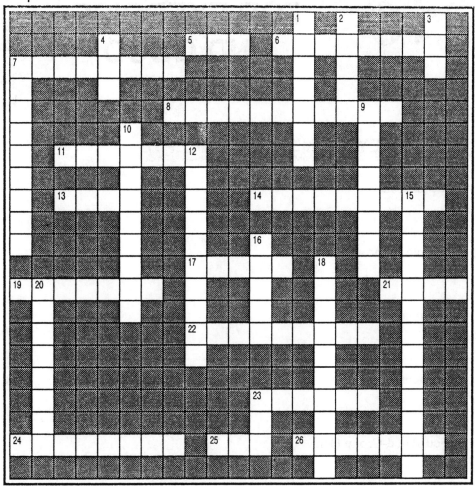

24 A specific recipe that is filed with the FDA is referred to as a standard of _____

25 Term describing a product that has been changed substantially within the prior 6 months

26 Term describing a product with no more than 35 mg of sodium/serving

DOWN

1 Term for carbon-containing compounds that has no legal meaning when applied to food labels

2 Refers to a single set of values recommended for nutritional requirements for each nutrient according to age and gender

3 Abbreviation for agency that regulates the advertising of food in the media

4 When a product has less than 0.5 g of fat per serving, it can be labeled "_____ free"

7 The term to describe adding vitamins and minerals to a food if they were previously missing

9 "No artificial _____" describes products free of the 33 coloring agents permitted in food products

10 Term describing a product devoid of all simple sugars

12 Term describing a product with no more than 40 kcal per serving

15 Term describing a product devoid of cholesterol

10 OPTIMAL NUTRITION FOR EXERCISE AND GOOD HEALTH

DEFINE KEY TERMS AND CONCEPTS

1. Optimal diet

2. Simple amino acids

3. Minimal level of fat

4. Prudent diet

5. Four-Food-Group Plan

6. Eating-right pyramid

7. Eat more, yet weigh less

8. Phosphatase

9. Hitting the wall

10. Staleness

11. Glycogen resynthesis

12. Glucose polymers

13. Drinks

14. Carbohydrate loading

15. Modified carbohydrate loading

16. Liquid meals

STUDY QUESTIONS

Recommended nutrient intake

What is the recommended percentage intake for fat, carbohydrate, and protein for active individuals?

Fat

Carbohydrate

Protein

Protein

For a physically active person, what is the recommended intake of dietary protein?

Preparations of simple amino acids

What is the most desirable form for dietary protein?

Lipid

What is the recommended lipid intake to promote good health? What types of lipids should be ingested?

Optimal lipid intake

Lipid type

Carbohydrate

What is the recommended form of dietary carbohydrate in terms of optimal nutrition? Why?

The Four-Food-Group Plan: the essentials of good nutrition

Outline the recommendations of the Four-Food-Group Plan.

The eating-right pyramid

Outline the recommendations of the eating-right pyramid.

Exercise and food intake

Caloric intake among athletes

Discuss whether athletes require a greater than average caloric intake.

Eat more, weigh less

Explain how it is possible for physically active people to actually eat more than the average person yet weigh less.

Diet and exercise performance

What is the macronutrient that eventually becomes depleted during long-term aerobic exercise?

Where is this macronutrient stored in the body?

Carbohydrate needs in intense training

Discuss what happens to the body's glycogen reserves during successive days of prolonged exercise.

Diet, glycogen stores, and endurance

What effect does modifying daily carbohydrate intake have on muscle glycogen and endurance exercise?

Sugary drinks before and during exercise: a wise solution?

During exercise

In what way can carbohydrate-containing drinks consumed during exercise affect performance?

What to drink?

Give a general recommendation for the composition of a carbohydrate drink.

Glucose feedings and water uptake

Identify a potential negative effect of drinking a concentrated carbohydrate-containing drink during exercise.

Before exercise

What effect does drinking a strong sugar solution 30 minutes prior to exercising have on performance?

<u>Effect</u>

<u>Reason</u>

Carbohydrate loading: a way to increase glycogen reserves

Outline the classic procedure for carbohydrate loading.

Negative aspects

Identify two potential negative aspects of the classic carbohydrate loading procedure.

1.

2.

Modified loading procedure

Outline the modified procedure for carbohydrate loading.

The precompetition meal

  High protein is not the best choice

    Give three reasons why a high protein pre-event meal is not desirable.

        1.

        2.

        3.

Liquid meals

    List two advantages of liquid feedings prior to competition.

        1.

        2.

PRACTICE QUIZ

MULTIPLE CHOICE

1. Drinking carbohydrate-containing beverages during exercise appears to be beneficial to performance:
   a. only at work level above 30% of maximum
   b. only at work levels above 60% of maximum
   c. only during sprint events
   d. by facilitating fluid uptake by the body

2. The common practice of consuming liquids, powders, or pills of predigested protein is ineffective because:
   a. amino acids are not required for muscle synthesis
   b. proteins are absorbed as di- and tripeptide molecules as well as in simple amino acid form
   c. excess dietary proteins cause muscle atrophy
   d. b and c

3. Fructose has been proposed to provide an advantage over glucose or sucrose for pre-event feedings because:
   a. fructose contains more energy per unit weight
   b. fructose is absorbed into the bloodstream more rapidly and thus is readily available for energy
   c. fructose does not trigger the release of cortisol
   d. fructose does not trigger the release of insulin
   e. a and d

4. Ingesting a solution of polymerized glucose during exercise could be beneficial because it would:
   a. reduce the osmolarity of the ingested fluid, thereby retarding fluid replacement
   b. increase the osmolarity of the ingested fluid thereby facilitating fluid replacement
   c. reduce the osmolarity of the ingested fluid thereby facilitating fluid replacement
   d. none of the above

5. Which of the following are TRUE statements:
   a. The liver's uptake of alanine during exercise exceeds that of all other amino acids
   b. Fatty acids serve as a source for synthesizing glucose
   c. The capacity to perform high intensity aerobic exercise is increased about 3 times when the diet is changed from carbohydrate-poor to carbohydrate-rich
   d. a and c
   e. all of the above

FILL-IN

1. The RDA for protein is _____ grams of protein per kg of body mass.

2. Lipid intake should not exceed _____ % of total calorie intake.

3. An active person should consume about _____ % of total caloric intake from carbohydrates.

4. _____ provides the predominant macronutrient fuel during low to moderate exercise.

5. _____ is a term to describe the feelings associated with a depletion of glycogen stores during exercise.

TRUE / FALSE

_____ 1. Except for total caloric intake, daily requirements for proper nutrition are similar for both the active person and the competitive athlete.

_____ 2. Endurance athletes require an increased dietary requirement of vitamins and minerals.

_____ 3. Protein intake above the RDA may place added strain on liver and renal function.

_____ 4. Active men and women eat more than sedentary people yet maintain a lower body weight.

_____ 5. If a solution of water and glucose is ingested at regular intervals during exercise, blood glucose will peak and then rapidly fall, causing the athlete to prematurely "hit the wall."

Chapter 10

ACROSS

4 Diet and exercise that "packs" muscle glycogen is termed carbohydrate _____

5 A diet where nutrient intake meets the needs for adequate tissue repair maintenance, and growth

6 This plan (3 words) for prudent eating emphasizes grains, vegetables, and fruits and de-emphasizes protein, lipids, and dairy products

7 Fifteen to 25 g daily of this macronutrient is probably a ____ ____ ____ ____ intake

11 Enzyme that reconverts glycogen to glucose

13 A popular 3-word term describing extreme difficulty exercising when carbohydrate reserves are low

14 Drinks containing glucose _____ counter the negative effects of simple sugar molecules on gastric emptying

15 Many of the negative aspects of classic carbohydrate-loading can be eliminated by following this less stringent plan

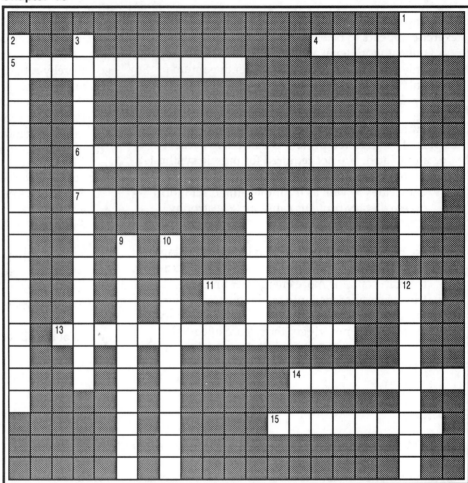

DOWN

1 Commercially prepared high-carbohydrate meals in this form are a practical pre-event feeding

2 Nutrition plan (4 words) utilizing 4 food categories and recommended number of servings

3 Chemically "predigested" proteins in this form are of no benefit to exercise or muscle building

8 Many physically active people can actually _____ _____ yet weight less

9 For fluid replacement, the optimal "_____ _____" should probably contain no more than 8% carbohydrate

10 After long-term exercise, at least 48 hours are required to allow for glycogen _____

12 A physiologic state of fatigue where continued hard training becomes progressively more difficult

11 ENERGY FOR EXERCISE

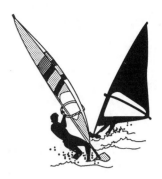

DEFINE KEY TERMS AND CONCEPTS

1. Biologic work

2. Energy

3. Adenosine triphosphate

4. Adenosine diphosphate

5. Aerobic

6. Anaerobic energy release

7. Creatine phosphate

8. Chemical energy

9. Glycolysis

10. Acetyl CoA

11. Mitochondria

12. Krebs cycle

13. Variations in body size on oxygen uptake

14. Oxygen uptake

15. Steady state

16. Maximal oxygen uptake

17. Inherited factors on aerobic capacity

18. Lactic acid

19. Lactate

20. Blood lactate threshold

21. Fast-twitch muscle fiber

22. Slow-twitch muscle fibers

23. Recovery oxygen uptake

24. Oxygen deficit

25. Lactic acid removal

Energy production in the body

  The energy currency, adenosine triphosphate

    What is the chemical make-up of ATP?

    What is the chemical make-up of ADP?

Aerobic and anaerobic energy release

    Discuss the basic difference between aerobic and anaerobic energy release.

The energy reservoir: creatine phosphate

    Draw the chemical reactions for the resynthesis of ATP from CP.

    Why is CP considered the "reservoir" of high energy phosphate?

Energy from food

What is the body's single purpose for the catabolism of its stores of carbohydrate, protein, and lipid?

List three reasons why glucose breakdown is a good example of energy release and transfer at rest and during exercise.

    1.

    2.

    3.

Anaerobic energy from food

Outline the chemical reactions in the breakdown of glucose in glycolysis.

Aerobic energy from food

Why are the mitochondria considered the powerhouses of the cell?

Describe the phase 1 and phase 2 chemical reactions of aerobic metabolism. (HINT: refer to Figure 11-7 in your textbook.)

Phase 1

Phase 2

Diagram the various pathways of energy metabolism for lipids, carbohydrates, and proteins. (HINT: refer to Figure 11-5 in your textbook.)

Lipids   Carbohydrates   Proteins

Oxygen uptake during exercise

Draw the curve for oxygen uptake during 10 minutes of moderate jogging exercise. Indicate the area of oxygen deficit and the point of steady state. (HINT: refer to Figure 11-8 in your textbook.)

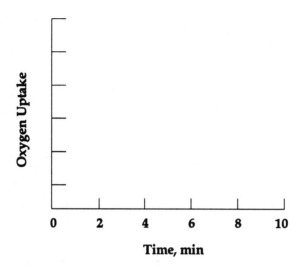

How would you express the oxygen uptake in relation to body mass for an individual who weighed 85 kg and consumed 2.0 liters of oxygen per minute during jogging?

There are many levels of steady-state

Explain why steady-state exercise for an endurance athlete could be exhausting for an untrained person.

Maximal oxygen uptake

Draw the curve that illustrates the oxygen uptake during a run up progressively steeper hills. Why does the oxygen uptake plateau or level off at the more extreme exercise levels?

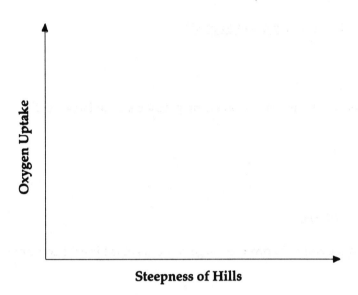

Define the term "maximum oxygen uptake".

List the average values (ml/kg/min) for max VO_2 for sedentary and endurance trained men and women.

	<u>Men</u>	<u>Women</u>
<u>Sedentary</u>		
<u>Endurance</u>		

Is fitness capacity inherited?

What is the impact of heredity on fitness capacity?

Lactic acid

> In terms of exercise metabolism:

>> <u>What is lactic acid?</u>

>> <u>Under what conditions is lactic acid formed?</u>

An important metabolic option

> During exercise, what is the advantage of converting pyruvic acid to lactic acid?

Training enhances lactate-forming tolerance

> In what activities would the ability to produce large amounts of lactic acid account for superior performance?

Blood lactate accumulation during exercise

> Illustrate the relationship between oxygen uptake and blood lactate accumulation during exercise of progressively increasing intensity in endurance trained and untrained individuals. (HINT: refer to Figure 11-12 in your textbook.)

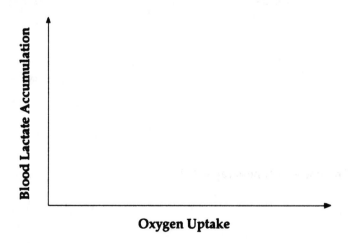

What is meant by the term "blood lactate threshold"?

Fast- and slow-twitch muscle fibers

List two characteristics of fast-twitch or Type II muscle fibers.

1.

2.

List two characteristics of slow-twitch or Type I muscle fibers.

1.

2.

Some questions concerning muscle fiber types

What are the differences in percentage distribution in muscle fiber type between the following groups:

	<u>Type I</u>	<u>Type II</u>
<u>Average person</u>		
<u>Successful endurance athlete</u>		
<u>Successful sprint athlete</u>		

In what ways can the metabolic capacity of fast- and slow-twitch fibers be changed by a specific exercise?

<u>Slow-twitch fibers</u>

<u>Fast-twitch fibers</u>

Recovery oxygen uptake

Draw the curves for oxygen uptake during recovery from light and heavy exercise. (Note the point at the end of exercise.)

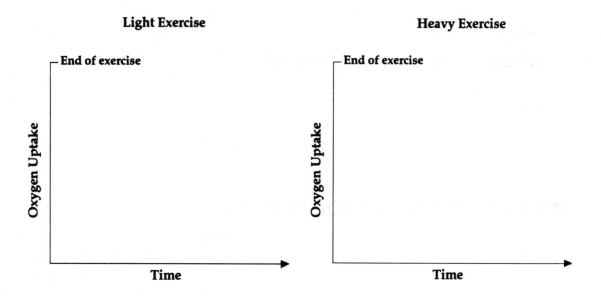

Light Exercise   **Heavy Exercise**

Recovery from moderate exercise

What is the purpose of the recovery oxygen uptake from moderate exercise?

Recovery from heavy exercise

What is the purpose of the recovery oxygen uptake from heavy exercise?

Keep active during recovery

Discuss some of the reasons for keeping moderately active during recovery from strenuous exercise.

The energy spectrum of exercise

Draw and label a diagram indicating the relative contributions of the sources of anaerobic and aerobic energy during maximal physical activities of various durations. (HINT: refer to Figure 11-15 in your textbook.)

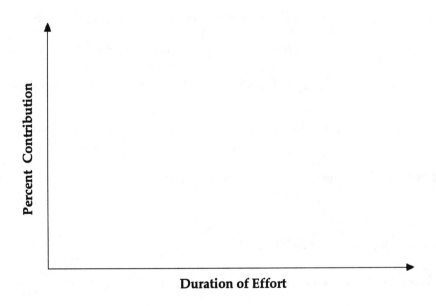

PRACTICE QUIZ

MULTIPLE CHOICE

1. During maximal exercise there is a point when oxygen uptake fails to increase despite an increase in the intensity of the work. This is known as:
    a. max CO_2
    b. maximum ventilation
    c. lactate threshold
    d. oxygen uptake
    e. maximum oxygen uptake

2. Lactic acid:
    a. is a metabolic waste product
    b. is not a metabolic waste product
    c. can cause anaerobic metabolism and O_2 debt
    d. can cause the Krebs cycle to stop if it isn't deaminated in the liver and voided in urine
    e. is formed from the union of three pyruvic acid molecules

3. Energy released from ATP and CP can sustain "all out" running and swimming for:
    a. 1 second
    b. 5 to 8 seconds

    c. 1 minute
    d. 4 minutes
    e. an unlimited time or until fatigue sets in

4. The chemical reactions of glycolysis:
    a. require oxygen
    b. do not require oxygen
    c. produce large amounts of ATP
    d. are essentially aerobic
    e. cause the release of nitrogen

5. During light exercise (40% of max $\dot{V}O_2$) the oxygen uptake curve rises sharply initially and then:
    a. flattens out and remains stable at steady state
    b. decreases sharply to match energy supply
    c. decreases toward the resting level after 3 minutes of exercise
    d. none of the above

FILL-IN

1. The energy-rich compound _____ is the "fuel" for all energy-requiring process of the cell.

2. ADP combines with _____ to reform the energy-rich compound ATP.

3. ATP production during _____ is important because it provides a rapid source of energy for muscular activity.

4. The freeing of _____ atoms during the Krebs cycle is one of the most important chemical events in the cell.

5. A person's maximum capacity to utilize oxygen during exercise is called the _____.

TRUE / FALSE

_____ 1. Heredity exerts only a small influence on max $\dot{V}O_2$.

_____ 2. The blood lactic acid level of sprint athletes in maximum exercise is the same as for untrained subjects.

_____ 3. The average percentage of slow-twitch muscle fibers in men and women is about 45 to 50%, but the variation among individuals is large.

_____ 4. The oxygen uptake in excess of the resting value consumed during recovery from exercise is called the oxygen deficit.

_____ 5. Lactic acid removal is accelerated by active aerobic exercise in recovery.

Chapter 11

ACROSS

1 Pyruvic acid + coenzyme A
3 Abbreviated term for aerobic capacity
5 Mechanical, chemical, and transport are all forms of this broad category of work
9 This twitch fiber has a high capacity for the aerobic production of ATP
10 $\dot{V}O_2$ in ml/kg/min adjusts for differences among individuals in this factor
11 _____ lactate becomes elevated during non steady-state exercise
12 All biologic work requires a continual supply of ____
14 Studies of identical twins indicate that a large component of max$\dot{V}O_2$ is _____
15 The buffered by-product of anaerobic carbohydrate metabolism
17 Metabolic pathway that forms H and CO_2 from Acetyl Co-A
18 Marathon runners possess a high maximum level of _____ _____
20 ATP splits into ADP and _____

DOWN

1 Energy releasing reactions that do not require oxygen
2 The elevated $\dot{V}O_2$ above rest after exercise is termed the _____ oxygen uptake
4 Referred to as the "powerhouse" of the cell
6 Pyruvic acid + 2 H
7 Break down of glucose to pyruvic acid
8 Heat energy is to an engine as _____ _____ is to the body
9 Metabolic condition where exercise energy requirements are met by aerobic metabolism
13 All biologic work requires a continual supply of _____
16 A characteristic of contraction to classify slow and fast muscle fibers
19 The hydrolysis of ATP forms _____

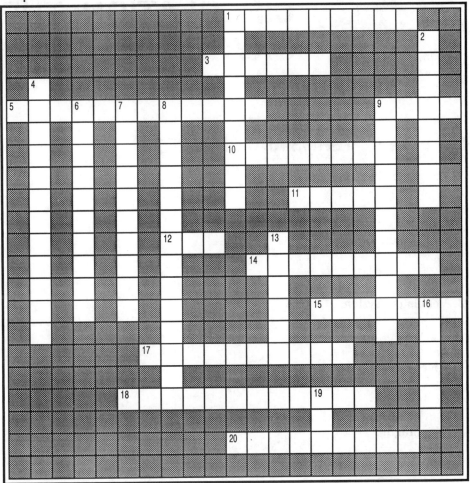

VENTILATION AND CIRCULATION: THE OXYGEN DELIVERY SYSTEMS

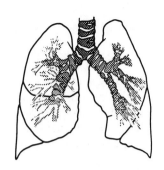

DEFINE KEY TERMS AND CONCEPTS

1. Oxygen delivery systems

2. Lung volume

3. Ventilatory system

4. Alveoli

5. Diaphragm

6. Inspiration

7. Expiration

8. Pulmonary ventilation

9. Glottis

10. Valsalva maneuver

11. Pressure differentials

12. Composition of centrifuged blood

13. Hematocrit

14. Hemoglobin

15. Anemia

16. Breathing oxygen-enriched gas

17. Pulmonary ventilation and oxygen uptake

18. Asthma

19. Exercise-induced asthmatic response

20. Post-exercise coughing

21. Effects of smoking

22. Heart

23. Arterial system

24. Capillaries

25. Veins

26. One-way flow of blood

27. Varicose veins

28. Milking action

29. Pulse

30. Blood pressure

31. Auscultatory method

32. Systole

33. Diastole

34. Sphygmomanometer

35. Hypertension

36. Heart failure

37. Stroke

38. Cardiac output

39. Heart rate

40. Stroke volume

41. Stroke volume of the athlete's heart

42. Maximum cardiac output and aerobic capacity

43. Patterns of cardiac enlargement

STUDY QUESTIONS

Pulmonary ventilation

Lung structure and function

Trace the pathway for inspired air as it moves through the major structures of the ventilatory system.

Mechanics of breathing

Outline the process of pulmonary ventilation in terms of ventilatory muscle action and alterations in thoracic dimensions during inspiration and expiration.

1. <u>Inspiration</u>

2. <u>Expiration</u>

Breathe normally during exercise

What effect does the Valsalva maneuver have on intrathoracic pressure and venous return?

<u>Intrathoracic pressure</u>

<u>Venous return</u>

Gas exchange in the lungs

Diagram the exchange of O_2 and CO_2 in the lungs and the subsequent diffusion of these gases in the tissues. Indicate the direction and magnitude of the changes that occur between rest and exercise.

Oxygen transport

What is the role of hemoglobin in oxygen transport?

Breathing oxygen-enriched gas

Explain why the breathing of oxygen-enriched gas mixtures following exercise is generally of no added benefit in terms of oxygen transport and recovery.

Pulmonary ventilation during exercise

Graph the relationship between pulmonary ventilation (vertical or Y-axis) and oxygen uptake (horizontal or X-axis) during successive increments in exercise intensity.

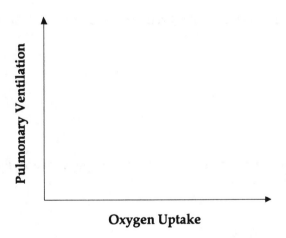

Why does overheating occur during heavy exercise?

The trained breathe less

What is the major difference in pulmonary ventilation between trained and untrained during submaximal exercise?

List two potential benefits of this difference to the trained individual.

    1.

    2.

Exercise and the asthmatic

What is the proposed mechanism by which exercise triggers an asthmatic response in susceptible individuals?

Cigarette smoking

In terms of pulmonary function, what is the short-term consequence of inhaling cigarette smoke?

Circulation

The cardiovascular system

List three important functions of the circulatory system during physical activity.

    1.

    2.

    3.

The heart

Sketch the details of the heart as a pump, indicating its chambers, valves, and major blood vessels entering and exiting it.

The arteries

In what way does the arterial system contribute to regulating blood distribution throughout the body?

The veins

Indicate how the following two factors facilitate the return of blood to the heart:

<u>Valves in veins</u>

<u>Muscle contractions</u>

Blood pressure

Indicate the meaning of the appearance and disappearance of sounds during blood pressure measurement.

What effect do straining exercises, such as heavy weight lifting, have on the following:

Resistance to blood flow in peripheral tissues

Blood pressure

Workload of the heart

Body inversion

What is the physiologic risk of body inversion?

Circulatory function in trained and untrained

The equation to determine the amount of blood pumped from the heart is:

Cardiac output = _____ X _____

Give representative values for cardiac output, heart rate, and stroke volume during rest and maximal exercise for both sedentary and highly trained young adults.

	Sedentary		Highly trained	
	Rest	Maximal exercise	Rest	Maximal exercise
Cardiac output				
Heart rate				
Stroke volume				

Close association between cardiac output capacity and maximal oxygen uptake

What is the relationship between maximum cardiac output and maximum aerobic capacity?

Why is it advantageous for an endurance athlete to possess a large maximum cardiac output?

Athlete's heart

How are different patterns of cardiac enlargement associated with different types of exercise training?

PRACTICE QUIZ

MULTIPLE CHOICE

1. If spread out, the lung tissue would cover a surface:
   a. equal to one-half a football field
   b. about 3 times the external surface of the person
   c. about 35 times the person's external surface
   d. equal to the external surface of a basketball
   e. b and d

2. The Valsalva maneuver:
   a. causes an abrupt and dramatic increase in pressure within the chest cavity
   b. causes an abrupt and dramatic decrease in pressure within the chest cavity
   c. leads to a prolonged increase in venous return
   d. is performed during endurance-type activities
   e. none of the above

3. Which of the following statements are TRUE about pulmonary ventilation in healthy people:
   a. During moderate exercise, ventilation increases linearly with oxygen uptake
   b. During submaximum exercise, ventilation is higher for the trained compared to the untrained
   c. During submaximum exercise, ventilation will be the same for the trained and untrained
   d. In strenuous exercise, ventilation cannot keep pace with the demand for oxygen
   e. a and b

4. Diffusion of gas in the lungs:
   a. is a passive procedure
   b. is an active procedure
   c. requires enzymes
   d. depends on the hemoglobin concentration

5. Which of the following are TRUE statements about Figure 12-6 in your textbook?
   a. Maximum ventilation is higher in the trained
   b. At a submaximal oxygen uptake the ventilation is lower for the untrained
   c. At an oxygen uptake of 45 ml/kg/min, the ventilation of the trained person is 90 l/min
   d. For both trained and untrained, ventilation decrease in relation to the oxygen demands

FILL-IN

1. The _____ are the microscopic, thin-walled terminal branches of the respiratory tract.

2. The major inspiratory muscle that makes an airtight seal that separates the lower chest from the abdominal cavity is the _____ .

3. The movement of gas molecules between the lungs and the blood and between the blood and the tissues occurs by the process of _____ .

4. The _____ are the blood vessels where nutrient and gas exchange takes place.

5. In healthy men and women at rest, the systolic blood pressure during a cardiac cycle of contraction and relaxation generally rises to _____ mmHg.

TRUE / FALSE

_____ 1. The lung volume of an average sized adult is generally between 4 and 6 liters.

_____ 2. For healthy individuals, maximal exercise does not fully tax an individual's capacity to breathe.

_____ 3. Diffusion in the healthy lung is so rapid that alveolar blood gas equilibrium takes only 5 seconds

_____ 4. The right side of the heart receives oxygenated blood from the lungs and pumps it into the aorta.

_____ 5. The ability of the exercise-trained heart to generate a large stroke volume is related to both a large left ventricular internal dimension and a more forceful ventricular contraction.

Chapter 12

ACROSS

1 A large maximum _____ output requires a large stroke volume
3 This 2-word term describes the flow of air into and out of the lungs
9 The process by which air leaves the lungs
10 Cardiac output = heart rate x _____ volume
11 Major inspiratory muscle
13 Concentration of red blood cells
15 Air _____ into and from the lungs occurs by pressure changes in the airways
18 Trained endurance athletes eject a large _____ of blood with each heart beat
19 Forced exhalation against a closed glottis
22 Muscular pump that propels blood throughout the body
24 _____ oxygen-enriched gas before exercising is of no benefit to subsequent exercise
25 A behaviorally-related habit that causes a variety of cardiopulmonary diseases
26 Contraction phase of cardiac cycle

DOWN

2 Valves in veins provide for the _____ _____ flow of blood
3 Chronically elevated blood _____ is a significant heart disease risk
4 Vital capacity is a _____ _____ that varies between 4 to 6 liters in an average-sized adult

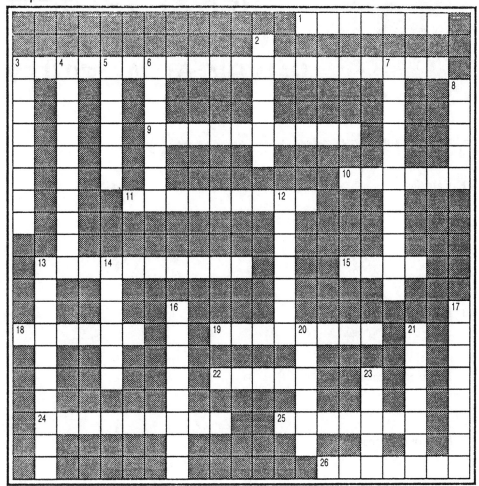

5 This gas moves across the alveoli into the blood
6 Terminal branches of the respiratory tract
7 The process by which air enters the lungs
8 _____ rate immediately after exercise is a good indication of exercise heart rate
12 Covers the trachea during swallowing
13 Iron-protein compound within red blood cell
14 Significantly low level of blood hemoglobin
16 Water loss and drying of the respiratory passages causes this following exercise
17 Relaxation phase of the cardiac cycle

20 An obstructive pulmonary disease that affects about 10 million Americans
21 Instrument called a _____ manometer measures blood pressure
23 Blood vessels that contain valves

13

ENERGY VALUE OF FOOD AND PHYSICAL ACTIVITY

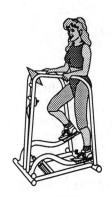

1. Calories

2. Kcal

3. Kilojoule

4. Bomb calorimeter

5. Heat of combustion

6. Digestive efficiency

7. Calorimetry

8. Human calorimeter

9. Indirect calorimetry

10. Open-circuit method

11. Closed-circuit method

12. Calorific equivalent for oxygen

13. Portable spirometer

14. Bag technique

15. Basal metabolic rate

16. Postabsorptive state

17. Dietary-induced thermogenesis

18. Gross energy expenditure

19. Net energy expenditure

20. Met

STUDY QUESTIONS

Energy contained in foods: calories

What is the difference between a calorie and a kilocalorie?

<u>Calorie</u>

<u>Kilocalorie</u>

Measurement of calories

Describe how the calories in food are measured.

Caloric value of foods

Heat of combustion

Give the heat of combustion for the three food macronutrients.

Food macronutrient	Heat of combustion
1.	
2.	
3.	

Digestive efficiency

How does the digestive efficiency affect the heat of combustion of each macronutrient?

<u>Carbohydrate</u>

<u>Lipid</u>

<u>Protein</u>

Calorie value of a meal

Compute the caloric value of a meal containing in 20 g of protein, 30 g of fat, and 75 g of carbohydrate.

<u>kcal (protein)</u>

<u>kcal (fat)</u>

<u>kcal (carbohydrate)</u>

<u>Total kcal</u>

A calorie is a calorie is a calorie ...

From an energy standpoint, why aren't 100 kcal of fat more fattening than 100 kcal of protein?

Heat produced by the body

   Direct calorimetry

Describe the technique of direct calorimetry in the measurement of human heat production.

Indirect calorimetry

Describe two methods of indirect calorimetry.

   1.

   2.

Calorific transformation for oxygen

In general, what is the acceptable value for human energy production for an oxygen uptake of 1.4 liter per minute?

Describe the following three procedures to measure oxygen uptake during physical activity.

   1. Portable spirometry

   2. Bag technique

   3. Computer instrumentation

Energy expenditure during rest and physical activity

List the three components of daily energy expenditure.

1.

2.

3.

Energy expenditure at rest: the basal metabolic rate

Describe three conditions for measuring the BMR.

1.

2.

3.

Influence of body size on resting metabolism

What is the preferred way to express the BMR to account for differences among men and women in body size?

Discuss two methods to estimate a person's daily energy expenditure.

1.

2.

Dietary-induced thermogenesis

The thermic effect of food contributes about what percentage of one's total energy expenditure?

Energy expenditure in physical activity

Discuss the differences between gross and net energy expenditure during physical activity.

<u>Gross</u>

<u>Net</u>

Energy cost of recreation and sport activities

How many kcal are expended playing volleyball for two hours for a person weighing 170 lb? (HINT: refer to Table 13-3 in your textbook.)

Effect of body mass

Draw the relationship between the energy expended during weight-bearing exercise and body mass. What does this relationship indicate?

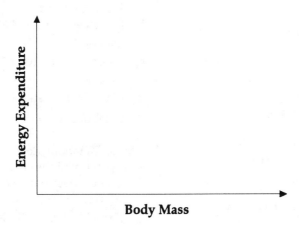

Average daily rates of energy expenditure

Discuss the primary factor that accounts for differences among people in their daily level of energy expenditure.

Classification of work

How is the MET level for a particular physical activity computed?

What are two factors that influence the difficulty of a task?

1.

2.

PRACTICE QUIZ

MULTIPLE CHOICE

1. Direct calorimetry involves:
   a. burning a food and measuring the amount of CO_2 liberated
   b. burning food and measuring the amount of heat liberated
   c. burning food and measuring the amount of O_2 consumed
   d. burning food and measuring the amount of H_2O produced

2. Foods that are relatively high in calories:
   a. generally are low in water content
   b. generally are rich sources of carbohydrate
   c. have a relatively low quantity of H atoms
   d. are usually high in fiber

3. What percent of the fat consumed in the diet is absorbed by the body:
   a. 80%
   b. 97%
   c. 90%
   d. 95%

4. One need only know the relationship between oxygen uptake and the liberation of energy to compute human energy expenditure because:
   a. 1 liter O_2 liberates 2.8 kcal when carbohydrate is metabolized
   b. 1 liter O_2 liberates 4.82 kcal when a mixed diet is metabolized
   c. 1 liter O_2 liberates 3.5 kcal when fat is metabolized
   d. 1 liter O_2 liberates 6.2 kcal when protein is metabolized

5. The Basal Metabolic Rate:
   a. is usually higher than the resting metabolism
   b. can be measured directly in a human calorimeter
   c. varies with age and gender
   d. is related to lean body mass
   e. b, c, and d

FILL-IN

1. A meal that is high in _____ will exert the greatest thermic effect.

2. If oxygen uptake during steady state swimming is 2.0 liters per minute, and resting $\dot{V}O_2$ is 0.30 l/min, for 10 minutes of exercise the net oxygen uptake is _____ liters.

3. If you gain lean body mass, your resting energy expenditure will _____ .

4, The _____ method of indirect calorimetry is the most practical for measuring energy expenditure during physical activity.

5. One's total daily energy expenditure is the sum of the energy required in _____ , _____ and _____ .

TRUE / FALSE

_____ 1. The average college-aged American woman expends about 2600 kcal per day.

_____ 2. In weight-supported exercise like stationary cycling, the energy cost of the exercise is closely related to body mass.

_____ 3. Generally, for most individuals the actual BMR is within $\pm$ 2% of the BMR predicted from age and gender.

_____ 4. If a person exercises at a steady-state oxygen uptake of 2.0 l/min in 30 minutes of exercise, 30 kcal will be burned.

_____ 5. A calorie is a unit of heat used to express the energy value of food or quantity of oxygen consumed.

Chapter 13

ACROSS

4 A value of 5.0 kcal is a general _____ transformation per liter of oxygen uptake

9 A unit of heat used to express the energy value of food

11 A unit of resting energy expenditure

12 Measurement of the body's heat production

13 This way of expressing exercise energy expenditure subtracts out the resting value

15 In the _____ technique of open-circuit spirometry, the subject breathes in ambient air and exhales into a collection device

16 The _____ - absorptive state is when a person has refrained from eating for at least 12 hours

17 This 3-word term relates to the heat measured when a food is burned

18 The _____ _____ average 97% for carbohydrates, 95% for lipids, and 92% for proteins

20 When the exercise energy value includes the resting value it is called the gross _____ expenditure

DOWN

1 This metabolic rate represents the body's minimum energy requirement in the waking state

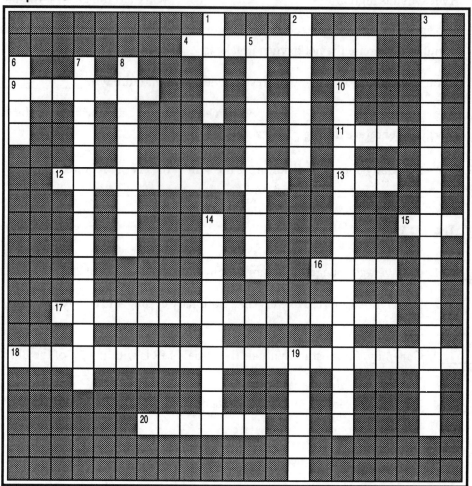

2 The increase in metabolism from digestion, absorption, and assimilation of nutrients is termed _____ induced thermogenesis

3 A technique to infer the body's heat production from oxygen uptake

5 The most widely used method of spirometry for indirect calorimetry

6 Abbreviation for amount of heat required to raise 1 kg of water by 1 degree C

7 A chamber for measuring the energy content of food

8 This international standard for energy is equivalent to 4.2 kilocalories

10 A chamber used to directly measure a person's heat production

14 This portable device is carried on the back for the indirect determination of energy expenditure

19 Subject rebreathes from a container of oxygen in _____ - circuit spirometry

PART 2

BODY COMPOSITION AND WEIGHT CONTROL

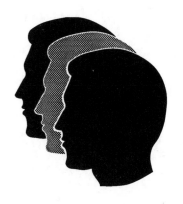

14 EVALUATION OF BODY COMPOSITION

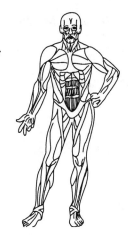

DEFINE KEY TERMS AND CONCEPTS

1. Dr. Albert Behnke

2. Overweight

3. Height-weight tables

4. Major structural components of the body

5. Reference man

6. Reference woman

7. Essential fat

8. Gender-specific fat

9. Storage fat

10. Lean body mass

11. Minimal weight

12. Oligomenorrhea

13. Amenorrhea

14. Menstrual irregularity

15. Lower cancer risk

16. Archimedes' principle

17. Specific gravity

18. Densities of fat and fat-free tissues

19. Hydrostatic weighing

20. Residual lung volume

21. Body density

22. Fatfold measurements

23. Frequently measured fatfold sites

24. Population specific

25. Generalized equations

26. Circumferences

27. Alternative indirect procedures

28. Ultrasound

29. BIA technique

30. CT and MRI

31. DEXA

32. Desirable body mass

STUDY QUESTIONS

Gross composition of the human body

List the three major structural components of the human body and their percentage as represented in the Reference man and Reference woman.

Structural components	Reference man	Reference woman
1.		
2.		
3.		

Reference man and Reference woman

Compare the body mass, stature, total fat, and storage and essential fat for the Reference man and woman.

	Reference man	Reference woman
Stature, cm		
Body mass, kg		
Total fat, kg		
Total fat, %		
Storage fat, kg		
Storage fat, %		
Essential fat, kg		
Essential fat, %		

Essential fat

What is the proposed function and location of essential fat and sex-specific essential fat in humans?

	Function	Location
Essential fat		
Sex-specific fat		

Storage fat

What is the proposed function and location of storage fat in humans?

Function

Location

Lean body mass (men)

Define and indicate the components that make up the lean body mass.

Definition

Components

What is the "healthy" lower level of percent body fat in males?

Minimal weight (women)

Define and indicate the components that make up the minimal weight in females.

Definition

Components

What is a "healthy" lower level of percent body fat in females?

Underweight and thin

What is precisely meant by the terms "underweight" and "thin"?

Underweight

Thin

Leanness, exercise, and menstrual irregularity

What is the association between menstrual irregularity and body fat?

Leanness is not the only factor

What is the lower limit of body fat believed necessary for maintaining normal menstrual function?

List four factors associated with menstrual dysfunction.

    1.   3.

    2.   4.

Delayed onset of menstruation and cancer risk

What is the relationship between delayed onset of menstruation and cancer risk and what is the proposed cause for this association?

<u>Relationship</u>

<u>Proposed cause</u>

Common laboratory methods to assess body composition

What are the two general procedures to evaluate body composition?

    1.

    2.

Direct assessment

Describe a major limitation of the direct method of body composition assessment in humans.

Indirect assessment

List three indirect procedures commonly used to assess body composition in humans.

1.

2.

3.

Archimedes' principle

What is Archimedes' principle of water displacement?

How is Archimedes' principle of water displacement used to evaluate body composition?

Determining body density

What is the approximate body volume of someone who weighs 50 kg when weighed in air, but only 2 kg when weighed submerged under water?

Computing percent body fat and mass of fat and lean tissue

Give the Siri equation to compute percent body fat from body density.

Compute percent body fat of a person whose body density is 1.0742 g/cc.

Give the equation and compute the fat mass for a person who weighs 63.4 kg and whose body fat is 10.8%.

    <u>Equation</u>

    <u>Fat mass</u>

Give the equation and compute the lean body mass of a person who weighs 63.4 kg with 6.85 kg of fat.

    <u>Equation</u>

    <u>Lean body mass</u>

Possible limitations

List two limitations of the generalized density values of 1.10 g/cc for fat-free tissue and 0.90 g/cc for fat tissue.

    1.

    2.

Measurement of body volume

Give the equation to determine body volume by hydrostatic weighing.

What procedure is used to determine the residual lung volume?

Why is residual lung volume assessed as part of the hydrostatic weighing procedure?

Fatfold measurements

What is the basis for the use of fatfold measurements to assess body fat in humans?

Describe the instrument and specific procedure to measure the thickness of subcutaneous fat.

Instrument

Procedure

List the five common sites for measuring fatfolds and their anatomic locations.

Sites	Anatomic location
1.	
2.	
3.	
4.	
5.	

Usefulness of fatfold scores

Discuss two ways to use fatfold scores in assessing body composition.

1.

2.

Fatfolds and age

What is the relationship between fatfolds and age?

Not for all people

Indicate a major drawback when using fatfolds in the assessment of body composition.

Girth measurements

Usefulness of girth measurements

List two advantages of girth measurements over fatfolds in assessing body fat.

1.

2.

Predicting body fat from girths

Compute the lean body mass for a 35 year-old woman who weighs 70.4 kg and whose girth measurements are as follows: abdomen = 82.6 cm; right thigh = 57.8 cm; right calf = 44.5 cm.

Other indirect procedures to assess body composition

Ultrasound

How is ultrasound used in the measurement of fat thickness?

Bioelectric impedance analysis (BIA)

What is the basic principle of BIA in assessing body composition? What factors can affect this measurement?

<u>Principle of BIA</u>

<u>Factors that affect BIA measurement</u>

Computed tomography (CT) and magnetic resonance imaging (MRI)

How is CT scanning useful in body composition assessment?

Discuss the use and advantage of MRI.

<u>Use</u>

<u>Advantage</u>

Dual-energy x-ray absorptiometry (DEXA)

In what ways are DEXA procedures useful in body composition assessment?

Average values for body composition

What are "average" values for percent body fat for young and older-aged adult males and females? (HINT: refer to Table 14-3 in your textbook.)

<u>Young males</u>   <u>Older males</u>

<u>Young females</u>   <u>Older females</u>

Representative samples are lacking

Discuss why it may not be necessarily "normal" for percent body fat to increase with increasing age.

Desirable body mass

Give the equation to compute "desirable body mass."

A 20-year old man weighs 89 kg and is 22% body fat. If the man begins a diet-exercise program and reduces his body fat to the desired 12% level, what will be his new body mass, and how much total fat mass will he have lost? (HINT: first compute desirable body mass, then compute desirable fat loss.)

<u>Desirable body mass</u>

<u>Desirable fat loss</u>

MULTIPLE CHOICE

1. Once underwater weight is known it is possible to compute all of the following except:
   a. body density.
   b. percent body fat
   c. lean body mass
   (d.) number and size of fat cells

2. Which of the following are FALSE statements:
   a. Highly trained male endurance athletes generally possess between 4 to 7% body fat
   b. Highly trained female endurance athletes generally posses between 14 to 18% body fat
   c. Low body fat levels in endurance-trained women are related to cessation of menses
   d. Even a moderate degree of obesity is related to an increased heart disease risk
   (e.) none of the above

3. The main limitation of height-weight tables is:
   a. they do not account for differences in bone structure
   b. they use body weight without considering age
   (c.) they give no indication of the composition of the body, especially fat and lean
   d. they are based on old normative data

4. According to Behnke's model for the Reference man and Reference woman:
   a. a woman may jeopardize her health if her body fat falls below 22%
   b. a man may jeopardize his health if his body fat falls below 8%
   (c.) the average quantity of essential fat for men is about 3% of body mass
   d. the average quantity of storage fat for women is about 26% of body mass
   e. none of the above

5. Very lean female athletes often experience secondary amenorrhea; this is indirect verification of Behnke's concept of:
   (a.) minimal weight
   b. storage fat
   c. energy drain
   d. lean body mass

FILL-IN

1. _____ is the amount of air remaining in the lungs following a maximal exhalation.

2. Body volume is usually measured by the procedure of _____ .

3. The existing prediction equations to calculate body composition from body density will tend to _____ the lean body mass when the equations are applied to blacks.

4. Body density is computed by dividing body mass by _____ .

5. _____ % body fat should be regarded as the lower range associated with maintenance of menstrual function.

TRUE / FALSE

_F_ 1. As body density increases, underwater weight decreases.

_F_ 2. The three major structural components of the body are body mass, lean body mass, and percentage fat.

_T_ 3. The error in predicting an individual's percentage body fat from fatfold or girth equations is generally within 2.5 to 4.0% fat units from the percent body fat determined by hydrostatic weighing.

_F_ 4. MRI is an abbreviation for multiple radiation imaging.

_F_ 5. Desirable body mass is computed as lean body mass minus percent fat desired.

Chapter 14

ACROSS

1 Body weight in excess of some average "weight-for-height"

5 Desirable fat _____ = present body mass minus desirable body mass

6 Two variables of body size used for determining ideal body weight from insurance company statistics

8 Greek mathematician who discovered the principle of water displacement

13 The Reference _____ is 15% body fat

14 _____ body mass for men is a body mass with a lower limit of 3% fat

16 Complete cessation of normal menses

18 Navy physician and foremost authority on body composition

20 This when divided by volume equals density

21 The _____ gravity is the ratio of its mass to the mass of an equal volume of water

22 Initials for technique to analyze body composition using electromagnetic fields

23 Value of 0.90 g/cc is considered the density of this tissue

24 The height-weight tables give no evaluation of _____ composition

25 Female athletes with delayed onset menstruation show a lower risk for this disease

26 For women, a lower limit of body mass that includes about 12 to 14% essential fat is termed _____ weight

DOWN

1 Irregular menstrual cycle

2 Fat depot required for normal physiologic functioning

3 The Reference _____ averages between 25 and 27% body fat

4 _____ equations take into consideration the influence of age when predicting body fat from fatfolds

5 The volume of air in this organ must be determined for precise measures of body volume

7 _____ weighing is a common technique to determine body volume

9 Fatfolds, ultrasound, hydrostatic weighing, and bioelectrical impedance are _____ methods to assess body composition

10 Initials for a technique commonly used to evaluate spinal osteoporosis

11 Fat depot that serves primarily as an energy reserve

12 Two-word term for additional component of essential fat characteristic in females

15 This menstrual abnormality increases the risk for osteoporosis at an early age

17 Mass per unit volume

19 Initials for indirect body composition technique that measures the body's resistance to an electrical current

21 The triceps, subscapula, and suprailiac are common _____ for measuring fatfolds

15 OBESITY

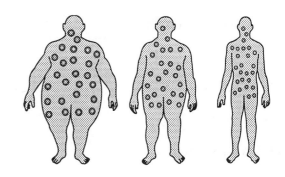

1. Reduced energy expenditure is a crucial factor

2. Obesity should be viewed as a disease

3. Risk of medical and health complications

4. Normal range of body fat

5. Standards for overfatness

6. Patterning of adipose tissue distribution

7. Android-type obesity

8. Gynoid-type obesity

9. Waist-to-hip ratio

10. Lipoprotein lipase

11. Fat cell hypertrophy

12. Fat cell hyperplasia

13. Dr. Jules Hirsch

14. Needle biopsy procedure

15. Phenotypic patterns

16. Adipose cellularity in obese and nonobese humans

17. Weight reduction

18. Weight gain

19. Development and growth of adipose tissue

20. Nutritional intervention

21. Exercise intervention

22. Spot reduction

Obesity: often a long-term process

On the accompanying figure, plot the trend for weight gain in young adult men and women as they age.

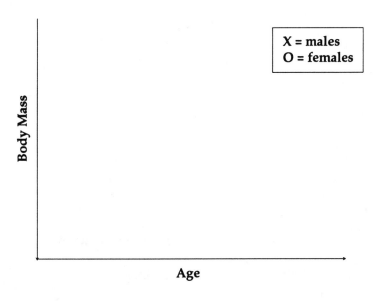

Not necessarily overeating

List five factors that predispose a person to excessive weight gain.

1.

2.

3.

4.

5.

Physical activity: an important component

Discuss whether the increase in body fat with age is more a function of physical inactivity than age itself.

Health risks of obesity

List five health risks that are related to obesity.

1.

2.

3.

4.

5.

Criteria for obesity: how fat is too fat?

Percent body fat as a criterion

Identify levels of percent body fat for establishing the beginning of obesity in adult men and women.

<u>Men</u>   <u>Women</u>

<u>Percent body fat</u>

Regional fat distribution as a criterion

Identify the two prevalent patterns of excessive fat distribution among obese men and women.

1.

2.

Give an objective standard for establishing male-pattern obesity.

Fat cell size and number

Indicate the two means of cellular development by which the body increases its quantity of adipose tissue.

1.

2.

Fat cell size and number in normal and obese adults

Give average values for fat cell size and fat cell number in obese and nonobese adults.

	<u>Obese</u>	<u>Nonobese</u>
<u>Cell size</u>		
<u>Cell number</u>		

Identify the major factor that differentiates the different gradations of obesity in terms of fat cellularity.

Fat cell size and number after weight reduction

What happens to fat cell size and fat cell number when adults lose weight?

1. <u>Fat cell size</u>

2. <u>Fat cell number</u>

Discuss the evidence concerning the possibility of "curing" fat cell hyperplasia.

Fat cell size and number after weight gain

What happens to fat cell size and fat cell number when adults gain a moderate amount of weight?

1. <u>Fat cell size</u>

2. <u>Fat cell number</u>

New fat cells may also develop

What happens to fat cell development during massive weight gain in adulthood?

Development of adipose cellularity

What happens to fat cell size during the different stages of human growth?

What happens to fat cell number during the different stages of human growth?

Modification of adipose cellularity

Nutritional influences

What are the effects of nutritional modification early in life on fat cell development in animals.

Exercise influences

What are the effects of regular exercise early in life on fat cell development in animals?

Spot reduction: does it work?

What effect does specific exercise have on localized fat loss?

Where on the body does fat loss occur?

PRACTICE QUIZ

MULTIPLE CHOICE

1. Which of the following statements are TRUE:
    a. With severe dietary restriction the actual number of fat cells decreases
    b. Increases in body fat in previously nonobese adults occur by filling existing fat cells rather than increasing cell number
    c. With further weight gain among the massively obese, new adipocytes may also develop
    d. a and c
    e. b and c

2. Adipocytes of newborn infants are about _____ the size of the average, nonobese adult:
    a. equal to
    b. double
    c. one-fourth
    d. one-tenth

3. According to the limited available data, fat cell number in humans probably increases significantly:
    a. during the first trimester of pregnancy
    b. during the last trimester of pregnancy
    c. during the first year of life

    d. during the fourth year of life
    e. b and c
    f. all of the above

4. Documented health risks of obesity include:
    a. coronary heart disease
    b. low blood pressure
    c. hyperthyroidism
    d. lymphatic cancer
    e. all of the above

5. For an average non-obese adult, a fat cell contains about _____ micrograms of fat:
    a. 0.9
    b. 28.0
    c. 0.1
    d. 0.6

FILL-IN

1. For children who are obese, the chances of becoming an obese adult are _____ times greater than for children who are not obese.

2. For women, a reasonable standard for "overfatness" is a percent body fat of _____ % or greater.

3. _____ is the enzyme associated with the regional regulation of body fat deposition.

4. Another term for fat cells is _____ .

5. Fat cells that store additional fat and increase in size are said to undergo _____ .

TRUE / FALSE

_____ 1. Approximately 110 million adult Americans are overweight and need to reduce body fat.

_____ 2. The average adult gains weight during middle age despite a progressive decrease in food intake.

_____ 3. Research indicates that there is no genetic link to one's susceptibility to becoming obese.

_____ 4. Among animals, early nutrition has no influence on the development of adult body fatness and adipose cellularity.

_____ 5. For the obese, weight loss is important for improving the blood lipid profile.

Chapter 15

ACROSS

1 Research indicates that a _____ _____ expenditure predisposes infants to gain weight

9 Male-pattern obesity

10 Excess body fat, not excess body _____ is the more important health risk

14 _____ for young adult men would be considered a body fat content in excess of 20%

16 Most adult weight gain is due to this change in adipocytes

17 _____ reduction does not occur in the abdominal area with repetitive sit-up exercise

18 When this is part of a weight loss program, more of the weight lost is fat

19 Enzyme that facilitates the uptake of fat by the adipocytes is _____ lipase

20 Six _____ _____ have been observed for body form in female obesity

DOWN

1 The NIH views even low levels of excess body fat to be a health _____

2 In light of the health risks of being overweight, health professionals now view obesity to be a _____

3 Extremes of obesity are more associated with this component of fat development

4 The _____ of fat on the body is largely influenced by regional activity of LPL

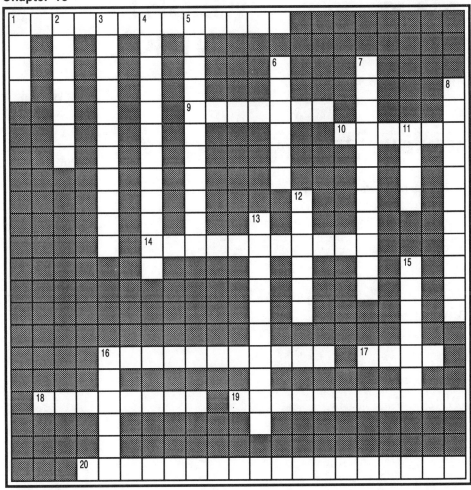

5 The _____ _____ for body fat in adults encompasses about plus or minus 1 unit of variation from the average value

6 The sampling of small amounts of fat from subcutaneous depots

7 A term for the significant increase in the number of fat cells

8 In animals, early _____ practices influence the development of body fat and adipose cellularity

11 It is probably not necessary for adults to _____ weight as they grow older

12 Type of fat patterning where fat accumulates in lower body regions

13 This ratio of fat patterning may be a more important indicator of health risk than total body fat

15 Synonym for fat tissue

16 Rockefeller University researcher who studied fat cellularity

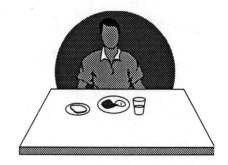

16 WEIGHT CONTROL

DEFINE KEY TERMS AND CONCEPTS

1. Ketogenic diets

2. Starvation diet

3. Very low calorie diet

4. High-protein diet

5. Energy balance equation

6. Set-point theory

7. Yo-yo effect

8. Effects of exercise on appetite and food intake

9. Weight cycling

10. Dose-response relationship

11. Acceptable limit of weight loss

12. Lean tissue is preserved

13. Ultimate "exercise prescription" for weight control

STUDY QUESTIONS

Dieting is not without risk

List three types of diet programs that have elicited strong opposition from responsible professional organizations.

1.

2.

3.

Ketogenic diets

What are ketogenic diets, what do they supposedly do, and are there any side-effects?

Ketogenic diet description

Supposed effects

Side effects

Starvation diets

List three underlying goals and two negative aspects of very low calorie diets (VLCD) .

Goals

1.

2.

Negative aspects

1.

2.

High-protein diets

Give two pros and two cons of high protein diets.

Pros

1.

2.

Cons

1.

2.

Maintenance of goal weight is a difficult task

What is the "bottom-line" concerning the success of long-term weight loss?

The energy balance equation

Write the energy balance equation.

Personal assessment of energy intake and energy output

Energy intake

List two reasons why it is important to keep records of food intake during a weight loss program.

1.

2.

Energy output

Unbalancing the energy balance equation

List three ways to unbalance the energy balance equation.

1.

2.

3.

Dieting to tip the energy balance equation

Describe a prudent approach to unbalancing the energy balance equation through diet only.

Set-point theory: a case against dieting

Explain the basis of the set-point theory.

Resting metabolism is lowered

Describe what generally happens to the basal metabolic rate when weight loss is attempted through dietary restriction only.

Weight cycling: going noplace fast

What is weight cycling and how does it affect one's chances for long-term weight control?

Weight cycling

Chances for success

Give a general recommendation for the composition of a weight-reducing diet.

How to select a diet plan

Give three guidelines for establishing a calorie-counting approach to weight loss.

1.

2.

3.

Well balanced but less of it

List two advantages of using a computerized diet and exercise plan for weight control.

1.

2.

Exercising to tip the energy balance equation

Explain how Americans can eat 5 to 10% fewer calories than they did 20 years ago, yet weigh an average 2.3 kg more.

Not simply a problem of gluttony

State the two arguments that oppose the use of exercise as a means for weight control.

1.

2.

Increased energy output worth considering

Effects of exercise on food intake

Discuss whether an increase in daily physical activity correspondingly increases daily food intake.

Effects of exercise on energy expenditure

In what way can exercise be effective for expending large numbers of calories?

Exercise is effective

List four factors to consider when designing an exercise program for weight control.

1.

2.

3.

4.

A dose-response relationship

Explain how weight loss relates to the amount of time a person exercises.

Is there a threshold energy expenditure for weight and fat loss? If so, what is it?

Regularity is the key

> When exercise is used in a program of weight loss, what is the recommended number of calories to be expended in each exercise session?

Diet plus exercise

> Why is the combination of exercise and diet the best approach to weight control?

Calculate the average daily caloric deficit to achieve a 20 lb fat loss in 20 weeks. Distribute the deficit equally between diet and exercise.

Total daily deficit

Deficit due to diet

Deficit due to exercise

Optimal duration of exercise plus diet program

What is the relationship between the caloric equivalent of weight lost and the duration of caloric restriction?

A radical approach: a challenge to exercise and health professionals

Describe a more radical approach to weight control using regular physical activity.

PRACTICE QUIZ

MULTIPLE CHOICE

1. If you burn 10 kcal/min you will have burned the calories in 1 pound of body fat in about:
   a. 500 minutes
   b. 6 hours
   c. 3 hours
   d. 200 minutes

2. When you lose weight by dieting only, body composition undergoes a:
   a. reduction in the size of individual fat cells
   b. reduction in the number of individual fat cells
   c. significant loss in total body fat, and an increase in lean tissue
   d. loss in both the fat and lean components
   e. a and d

3. Severe dieting is an ineffective approach to prudent weight loss because:
   a. it increases water retention
   b. more lean tissue is lost compared to the same caloric deficit created by a combination of exercise and moderate food restriction
   c. obese people do not eat in great excess so a true gluttony is often not the problem
   d. a and c
   e. all of the above

4. Which of the following statements are TRUE?
   a. When body weight is lost by either diet or exercise, almost all of the weight lost is fat
   b. Exercise is usually not an effective means for weight loss since it stimulates appetite
   c. For effective weight loss you should lose no more than 4 pounds per week
   d. The calorie cost of a marathon does not equal the calories in 1 pound of adipose tissue

5. The energy stored in a pound of body fat:
   a. is equal to 4500 kcal
   b. is sufficient to sustain most adults' BMR for one week
   c. provides the energy equivalent of an 85-mile run
   d. none of the above

FILL-IN

1. The three ways to unbalance the energy balance equation are _____, _____, and _____.

2. Long-term weight loss through dietary restriction generally is successful less than _____ percent of the time.

3. A caloric deficit of 3500 kcal created by diet or exercise is the equivalent to the calories in _____ lb of body fat.

4. Exercise enhances the conservation of _____ and the burning of _____ .

5. The rapid weight loss during the first few days of a caloric deficit is due primarily to the loss of _____ and _____.

TRUE / FALSE

_____ 1. Small variations in the percentage of carbohydrate, fat, and protein in a low-calorie, well-balanced diet do not make a difference in weight loss.

_____ 2. Diets that restrict water intake cause a greater weight loss but the extra weight lost is mostly water.

_____ 3. After several weeks on a low-calorie diet the caloric equivalent of each pound of weight lost is much greater than the caloric equivalent of the weight lost during the first week.

_____ 4. Maintaining adequate carbohydrate intake on a low-calorie diet helps to conserve lean tissue during weight loss.

_____ 5. Combining exercise with a low-calorie diet helps conserve the body's lean tissue during weight loss.

Chapter 16

ACROSS

4 A diet that stimulates the formation of acid by-products of incomplete fat breakdown
5 The important goal of dieting is to achieve fat loss, not simply _____ _____
8 Acronym is VLCD
12 This effect refers to repetitious bouts of dieting followed by subsequent weight gain
13 For weight loss, at least 3 days a week is a desirable _____ for exercising
14 Sixty minutes/day is a recommended _____ of exercise for weight loss
15 Rx for physical conditioning and training

DOWN

1 This approach to dieting greatly increases the chances for malnutrition and lean tissue loss
2 The most important step to weight loss is to do this to the energy balance equation
3 Proponents of this theory argue that the body physiologically tries to maintain a particular weight
6 There is little loss of _____ _____ when a weight loss diet contains adequate carbohydrate
7 This kind of diet has been associated with significant health risks, including death
9 Another term for the yo-yo effect in weight loss

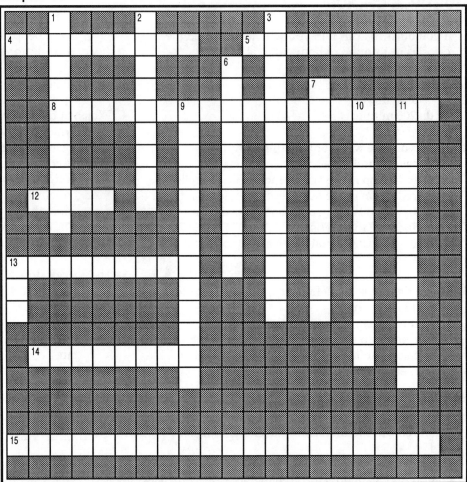

10 A direct _____ _____ relationship has been demonstrated between weight loss and the time spent exercising
11 A person is considered to be in _____ _____ when body weight remains stable over time
13 More of this is lost when weight loss is accompanied by regular exercise

17

MODIFICATION OF EATING AND EXERCISE BEHAVIORS

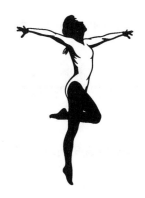

DEFINE KEY TERMS AND CONCEPTS

1. Behavior modification

2. Anorexia nervosa

3. Bulimia nervosa

4. Basic principles of behavior modification

5. Food cues

6. External factors influence eating behavior

7. Describe the various eating behaviors

8. Substitute behaviors

9. Techniques for gaining control over eating behaviors

10. TV watching and the prevalence of obesity

11. Time-in-motion analysis

12. Obese children are generally less active

13. Exercise behavior modification

14. Maximize exercise success

STUDY QUESTIONS

Eating behavior

List two important reasons why humans eat.

1.

2.

External cues

Describe the results of two studies that show how external factors influence eating behavior.

1.

2.

Modification of eating behavior

Describe the 1967 experiment for treating obesity by behavior modification techniques.

Describing the behavior to be modified

List seven items used to describe various eating behaviors and habits.

1.   5.

2.   6.

3.   7.

4.

Substituting alternative behaviors

List six examples of existing behaviors associated with eating and their replacement behaviors.

Existing behaviors   Replacement behaviors

1.   1.

2.   2.

3.   3.

4.   4.

5.   5.

6.   6.

List three techniques that can be used to gain control over existing eating habits.

1.

2.

3.

Other useful techniques

List 10 additional techniques that can be used to gain control over eating habits.

1.   6.

2.   7.

3.   8.

4.   9.

5.   10.

Provide positive reinforcement or rewards

List three long-term rewards or benefits for achieving weight loss through a planned program of eating behavior modification.

1.

2.

3.

Exercise behavior

  Modification of exercise behavior

    Compare the eating behaviors of obese and nonobese children.

      <u>Obese</u>

      <u>Nonobese</u>

    Compare the physical activity patterns of obese and nonobese children.

      <u>Obese</u>

      <u>Nonobese</u>

    What is a pedometer and how can it be used to modify physical activity behaviors?

    How does physical inactivity relate to the development of obesity?

  Describing the behavior to be modified

    Outline the first step in determining one's daily pattern of physical activity.

Substituting alternative behaviors

List five ways to replace sedentary activities with ones that are more physically demanding.

1.

2.

3.

4.

5.

Developing techniques to maximize exercise success

List five techniques to maximize the "fun" potential of exercise.

1.

2.

3.

4.

5.

Provide positive reinforcement or reward

Describe a way to provide positive reinforcement or reward for achieving success with exercise.

PRACTICE QUIZ

MULTIPLE CHOICE

1. The difference between hunger and appetite is that:
   a. appetite is related to physiological factors; hunger is not
   b. hunger is related to psychological factors; appetite is not
   c. hunger is socially "programmed" and genetically determined
   d. hunger is related to the body's need to supply food to sustain life
   e. appetite is related to the body's need to supply food to sustain life

2. Approximately how many times a month does the average American eat out at fast-food restaurants:
   a. 3
   b. 9
   c. 15
   d. 18
   e. 22

3. Which one of these techniques is not normally used to gain control over eating habits?
   a. make the act of eating food a ritual
   b. use larger dishes so the food appears smaller on the plate
   c. eat slowly; fight the urge to eat quickly by taking more time at meals
   d. cut food into smaller pieces
   e. chew food 12 to 15 times before swallowing

4. Time-in-motion studies of obese and normal-weight high school girls revealed differences for:
   a. participation in bowling, golf, watching TV
   b. total intake of carbohydrates and lipids
   c. total intake of fat-soluble vitamins
   d. participation in strenuous physical activities
   e. the levels of the hormones renin and pepsin

5. What is the most important consideration to increase energy expenditure on a long-term basis:
   a. enjoyment and success in physical activity
   b. exercise at a MET level equal to 4
   c. optimize the rate of energy hydrolysis
   d. conserve lean tissue
   e. stimulate oxidation of free-fatty acids

FILL-IN

1. Compared to obese individuals, lean individuals are characterized by healthy eating behaviors and an increased level of _____ .

2. A breakthrough was made in the treatment of obesity in 1967 when a psychologist reported the results of a one year program using _____ techniques to help individuals control their body weight.

3. Anorexia nervosa and _____ _____ are two common eating disorders.

4. Obese children are generally _____ active than leaner children.

5. A _____ is an instrument to assess physical activity involving walking and running.

TRUE / FALSE

_____ 1. Behavior modification techniques are used successfully in the treatment of anorexia nervosa.

_____ 2. Two reasons why people eat are (a) true hunger, and (b) the taste of food.

_____ 3. Daily events and psychological mood are unrelated to food itself and not likely to trigger the urge to eat.

_____ 4. Encouragement and positive reinforcement, in addition to self-discipline, must be built-in features of a successful weight control program.

_____ 5. The food intake of obese men and women is generally no greater than for people of normal body size.

Chapter 17

ACROSS

2 Important goal of behavior therapy to enable one to gain _____ over eating habits

4 Useful behavioral strategy to substitute _____ that are undesirable with more desirable ones

5 Psychological therapy to identify, control, and modify undesirable behaviors so they become desirable

7 The basic _____ of behavior modification include four strategies for success

8 This form of analysis (3 words) traces the actual time a person spends in daily physical activity

9 Sight, smell, and visual appearance of food are examples of _____ factors that affect eating behavior

11 Weight gain is often associated with a combination of faulty activity behaviors and poor _____ _____

DOWN

1 Behavior therapy is also called behavior _____

3 This condition is often related to a low caloric output rather than an excessive caloric intake

5 Eating disorder involving binge eating and subsequent purging of ingested food

6 Eating disorder where the person fails to maintain body mass at a "safe" level

10 An important step in eating behavior modification is to identify and then eliminate undesirable _____ cues linked to excessive caloric intake

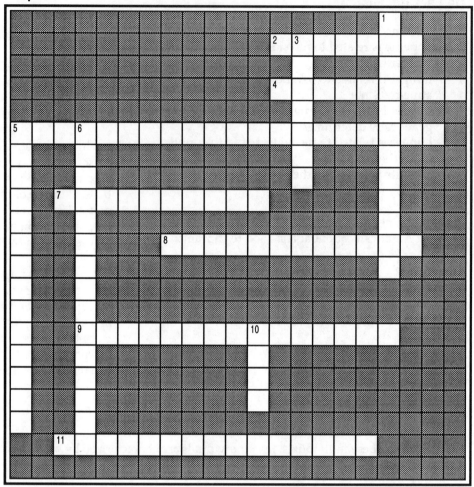

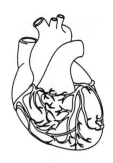

PART 3

PHYSIOLOGIC CONDITIONING FOR TOTAL FITNESS

DEFINE KEY TERMS AND CONCEPTS

1. Total fitness

2. Physiologic conditioning

3. Overload principle

4. Progressive overload

5. Training specificity principle

6. Individual difference principle

7. Reversibility principle

8. "Coronary prone"

The concept of total fitness

List four important components of total fitness.

1.

2.

3.

4.

General principles of physiologic conditioning

Briefy discuss and give examples of the following as they relate to exercise training and physical fitness:

Overload principle

Specificity principle

Individual difference principle

Reversibility principle

A word of caution before you begin

What is the major purpose for a medical check-up before beginning an exercise program?

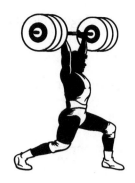

18 CONDITIONING FOR MUSCULAR STRENGTH

1. Concentric contraction

2. Eccentric contraction

3. Isometric contraction

4. Progressive resistance exercise

5. Isometric strength training

6. Limitations of isometric training

7. Benefits of isometric training

8. Specificity of resistance training

9. Isokinetic resistance training

10. Sticking point

11. Psychological factors

12. Muscular factors

13. Hypertrophy

14. Hyperplasia

15. Gender characterization of muscular strength

16. Gender difference in the response to resistance training

17. Testosterone

18. Metabolic stress of standard resistance exercises

19. Cardiorespiratory demands of circuit resistance training

20. Preliminary warm-up exercise

21. Stretching exercises

22. The lower back is susceptible to injury

23. Sufficient overload for improvement

Different forms of muscular contraction

Define and give examples of the three types of muscular contraction.

<u>Type</u>   <u>Example</u>

1.

2.

3.

Types of resistance training

Weight training: dynamic exercise

Outline the general scheme for progressive resistance exercise (PRE) training used by researchers in rehabilitation medicine following World War II.

Summarize the research findings concerning the recommended number of sets and repetitions for PRE training.

<u>Recommended sets</u>

<u>Recommended repetitions</u>

Isometric training (static exercise)

Discuss whether isometric training is desirable for improving performance in most sport activities.

List three limitations and two benefits of isometric resistance training.

Limitations

1.

2.

3.

Benefits

1.

2.

Which are better, static or dynamic methods?

"In all likelihood, neither static nor dynamic resistance training methods are inherently superior." Discuss.

What role does the nervous system play in the specificity of the training response to resistance exercises?

Isokinetic training

What is unique about isokinetic training in comparison to other forms of resistance training?

"With standard weight-lifting exercises the weight lifted can be no heavier than the force-generating capacity of the muscle (or muscles) at the weakest point in the range of motion." Discuss.

Adaptations with strength training

What are the six factors that impact on the development and maintenance of muscle mass?

1.   4.

2.   5.

3.   6.

Factors that modify the expression of human strength

Psychological factors

In what way do neural (psychological) factors contribute to strength improvement in the early phase of resistance training?

Muscular factor

List three of the so-called "physical factors" that ultimately determine a person's strength capacity.

1.

2.

3.

List six favorable physiologic adaptations that occur in response to resistance training.

1.   4.

2.   5.

3.   6.

Muscular strength of men and women

Discuss the gender differences in upper- and lower-body muscular strength.

Upper-body strength

Lower-body strength

Strength training for women

Muscular strength and hypertrophy

Summarize the research concerning muscular hypertrophy in women in response to resistance training.

Metabolic stress of resistance training

Isometric and weight-lifting exercise

In terms of total energy expended during a workout, how would you classify standard training programs of isometric and weight-lifting exercise?

Circuit resistance training

How have standard resistance exercise training programs been modified to increase the metabolic and cardiovascular demands of the workout?

Organizing a resistance training program

The warm-up

What is the purpose of the pre-exercise warm-up?

How should stretching exercises to improve joint flexibility be performed?

The lower back

What are the two primary fitness factors that protect against lower-back pain?

1.

2.

Describe the proper technique for performing a sit-up.

Selecting the proper weight

Discuss the amount of resistance and number of exercise repetitions when beginning a muscle strengthening exercise program.

Resistance

Repetitions

As the muscle-strengthening program progresses, what modifications should be made in the number of repetitions to enhance the effectiveness of the overload?

Six steps in planning the workout

Outline the six important steps to be followed when formulating a program to develop muscular strength.

1.

2.

3.

4.

5.

6.

PRACTICE QUIZ

MULTIPLE CHOICE

1. For the three types of muscular contractions in Figure 18-1 which of the following are TRUE?
   a. Illustration A shows an eccentric contraction: the muscle shortens to overcome the external resistance and cause movement
   b. Illustration B shows an isometric contraction: the external resistance exceeds the muscular force and the muscle lengthens with tension.
   c. Illustration C shows a concentric contraction force is generated with no shortening or movement
   d. Illustration A shows an isokinetic contraction: the muscle shortens to overcome external resistance and cause movement
   e. none of the above

2. The most effective approach to progressive resistance exercise training is to:
   a. keep the resistance constant and progressively increase the number of repetitions of exercise
   b. keep the repetitions between 3 and 9 RM and increase resistance as strength improves
   c. keep the resistance and repetitions constant and progressively increase the number of sets
   d. keep the repetitions between 12 and 20 RM and increase resistance as strength improves

3. The data in Figure 18-2 data support which type of training:
   a. weight lifting using concentric contraction
   b. weight lifting using eccentric contraction
   c. isometric training at a knee angle of 75°
   d. isometric training at a knee angle of 135°
   e. isokinetic training

4. Which of the following statements are TRUE about resistance training and strength development:
   a. The greatest increases in isometric strength occur when strength is measured in the exact position as the isometric training
   b. Dynamic resistance training produces greater improvement in muscular strength compared to isometric training
   c. Isokinetic resistance training produces greater improvement in muscular strength compared to isometric or dynamic training
   d. Strength improvement in one form of training is equal when the same muscles are evaluated in another form of training

5. Strength improvement in the latter phase of a resistance training program is largely due to:
   a. a significant hyperplasia of the muscle fibers
   b. learning and skill factors
   c. neural facilitation and removal of inhibition
   d. adaptations in the contractile structures
   e. a and d

FILL-IN

1. _____ -twitch muscle fibers show the greatest hypertrophy in response to resistance training.

2. For upper body strength, the average woman exhibits about _____% of the strength of the average male.

3. _____ is a form of resistance training that does not stress heavy muscular overload to improve fitness.

4. _____ is a form of resistance training that produces maximum force capacity at a pre-set speed.

5. Figure 18-9 shows that rapid strength changes in the early phase of resistance training are largely the result of _____ adaptations.

TRUE / FALSE

_____ 1. Traditional resistance training is of limited value for weight loss because total calorie expenditure is low.

_____ 2. Research indicates that women show little or no muscular hypertrophy in response to resistance training.

_____ 3. Physiologic conditioning for men is basically the same as for women regardless of age.

_____ 4. Performing one set of a resistance exercise is as effective as performing two or three sets.

_____ 5. Barbells, dumbbells, and isometrics are inherently superior to isokinetics for strength development.

Chapter 18

ACROSS

1 System of static resistance training popularized in the mid 1950s

4 Hormone that exerts an anabolic effect

6 The fact that isometric strength development is joint-angle specific is one of the _____ of this training

7 Enlargement of individual muscle fibers

9 CRT significantly increases the metabolic _____ of resistance training

11 First word in the abbreviation PRE

13 Muscle shortens while developing tension

14 Strength developed in one mode does not always transfer when measured in another mode illustrates this training principle

15 The weakest point in the range of motion is often termed the "sticking _____"

16 Muscle contraction where maximum force is generated throughout movement at a preset, fixed speed

18 Usually is the initial component of a workout

19 This demand is relatively low with standard resistance training

DOWN

2 Although psychological factors play a role, the ultimate limit to strength development is probably set by _____ _____

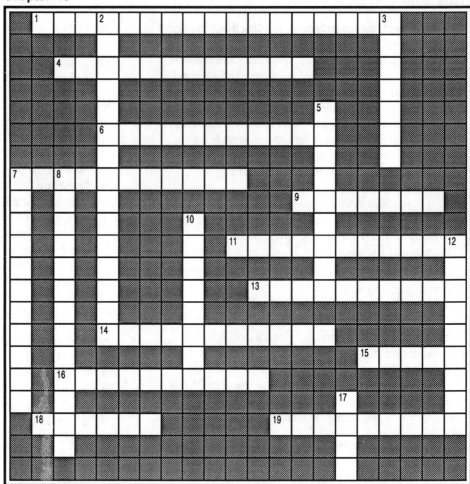

3 Differences in body size and composition mainly account for the large absolute strength differences between the _____

5 Length of muscle remains constant while generating force

7 Increase in the number of individual muscle fibers

8 These factors probably account for the rapid increase in strength early in resistance training

10 Weight training is considered a dynamic form of progressive resistance _____

12 Muscle lengthens while developing tension

17 Area of body susceptible to injury with improper resistance training

19

CONDITIONING FOR ANAEROBIC AND AEROBIC POWER

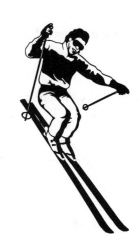

1. Anaerobic energy system

2. Aerobic energy system

3. Anaerobic-to-aerobic continuum

4. The phosphate pool

5. Overload of the phosphate pool

6. Training of the lactic acid system

7. Lactate stacking

8. Step test

9. Pattern of heart rate recovery

10. Queens College Step Test

11. Measurement of heart rate

12. Estimate of maximal oxygen uptake

13. Aerobic capacity classifications

14. Tecumseh Step Test

15. Goals of aerobic conditioning

16. Five factors influence aerobic conditioning

17. Initial fitness level

18. Training frequency

19. Duration of daily workout

20. Intensity of training

21. Threshold for aerobic improvement

22. Conversational exercise

23. Recommendations of the American College of Sports Medicine

24. Specificity of training

25. "Big muscle" activities

26. Guidelines for initiating aerobic training

27. Venous pooling

28. Individualize exercise training

29. Train at a percentage of maximal oxygen uptake

30. Train at a percentage of maximum heart rate

31. Age-predicted maximum heart rates

32. Training sensitive zone

33. Maximum heart rate for swimming

34. Rating of perceived exertion

35. Continuous exercise training

36. Interval exercise training

37. Exercise interval

38. Relief interval

39. Fitness maintenance

40. Exercise and pregnancy

STUDY QUESTIONS

Energy for exercise: it's the blend that's important

Outline the relative percentage involvement of the ATP-CP, lactic acid, and aerobic energy transfer systems during "all-out" exercise of varying durations.

	ATP-PC	Lactic acid	Aerobic
Up to 10 seconds			
Up to 90 seconds			
Between 2 and 4 minutes			
Beyond 4 minutes			

Identify the predominant energy system involved in the following:

	Energy system
100-yd dash	
880-yd run	
10-km (6.2 mi) run	

The anaerobic energy system

The phosphate pool

Outline an exercise program to overload the capacity of the high energy phosphates for back-stroke swimming.

Lactic acid

Outline an exercise program to overload the capacity of the lactic acid system for bicycle exercise.

The aerobic energy system

Aerobic conditioning

List three terms that describe the component of fitness required for sustained muscular activity.

1.

2.

3.

A useful method to evaluate cardiovascular capacity

What is the rationale for the use of the step test to evaluate the efficiency of the cardiovascular response to aerobic exercise?

Outline the method for administering the Queens College Step Test in terms of:

Bench height

Stepping cadence

Stepping duration

Period of pulse measurement

How can the measurement of recovery pulse rate be used to estimate a person's heart rate during exercise?

Factors that affect aerobic conditioning

List the two major goals of an aerobic training program.

1.

2.

Discuss how the following factors influence a person's response to aerobic training:

Initial level of cardiovascular fitness

Frequency of training

Duration of training

Intensity of training

Specificity of training

In terms of the threshold exercise intensity required to produce an aerobic training response, indicate the following:

Percent of max $\dot{V}O_2$ required

Percent of maximum heart rate required

Actual exercise heart rate for a college-aged male or female

Specificity of training

Outline the findings of two research projects that have shown a significant specificity in the aerobic response to training.

1.

2.

Developing an aerobic conditioning program

Discuss the purpose of the warm-up and cool-down periods in a training session.

Warm-up

Cool-down

Determining the training intensity

Compute the age-predicted maximum heart rate for a 54-year-old female.

What is her recommended threshold exercise heart rate to stimulate improvement in aerobic fitness?

What is meant by the term "training sensitive zone"?

Compute the 70% and 85% maximum heart rate exercise training limits for a 35-year-old male.

70% max HR

85% max HR

Adjust for swimming and other upper body exercises

What adjustment needs to be made in the "training sensitive zone" heart rates when swimming or other upper body exercise is used in training?

Is less intense exercise effective?

If aerobic exercise is performed at a level somewhat below the 70% threshold heart rate level, what adjustment should be made in the workout to assure a training effect?

Train at a perception of effort

Indicate how the "rating of perceived exertion" (RPE) can be used to establish the appropriate exercise intensity for aerobic training.

Continuous vs. intermittent aerobic conditioning

Continuous exercise training

Describe a continuous exercise training program.

Interval exercise training

What is meant by interval exercise training?

Why can exercise intensities that would rapidly fatigue a person if performed continuously be performed intermittently with the proper spacing of exercise-relief intervals?

Maintaining aerobic fitness

Discuss the role of exercise frequency, duration, and intensity if your goal is to <u>maintain</u> the improved level of aerobic fitness brought about by training.

<u>Frequency</u>

<u>Duration</u>

<u>Intensity</u>

Exercising during pregnancy

Summarize the effects of exercising during pregnancy on:

Energy cost

Fetal blood supply

Outcome (birth)

PRACTICE QUIZ

MULTIPLE CHOICE

1. Based on the information in Figure 19-1, which of the following statements are TRUE:
   a. All-out exercise up to 10-sec places a large demand onthe anaerobic breakdown of glucose
   b. All-out exercise of 2 minutes places a large demand on the anaerobic energy pathways
   c. One play in football is powered almost exclusively by energy from high energy phosphates
   d. The longer the exercise duration, the greater the involvement of the aerobic energy system
   e. b, c, and d

2. The most effective training of the short-term lactic acid energy system occurs with:
   a. one bout of all-out exercise of at least 3 minutes duration to the point of exhaustion
   b. repeat bouts of up to 1 minute of all-out exercise with 3 to 5 minutes of recovery
   c. repeat bouts of 5 to 10 seconds of all-out exercise with 3 to 5 minutes of recovery
   d. continuous exercise of 20 min with heart rate in the upper range of the "training sensitive zone"

3. Use of repetitive all-out exercise interspersed with recovery illustrates:
   a. continuous exercise training
   b. isokinetic exercise training
   c. dynamic exercise training
   d. interval exercise training
   e. none of the above

4. The following terms are used to indicate the body's capacity to generate ATP aerobically:
   a. maximum oxygen uptake
   b. aerobic capacity
   c. endurance fitness
   d. cardiovascular fitness
   e. a and c
   f. all of the above

5. For individuals of the same age, a low heart rate during and in recovery from a step test indicates a:
   a. large stroke volume of the heart
   b. relatively high level of aerobic capacity
   c. relatively high level of endurance fitness
   d. high level of hemoglobin in the blood
   e. a, b, and c

FILL-IN

1. If exercise _____ is maintained, the frequency and duration of training can be reduced considerably without any decrement in aerobic capacity.

2. Maximum performance of all-out exercise of up to 90 seconds' duration depends predominantly on one's capacity for _____ energy metabolism.

3. In the Tecumseh Step Test the bench height is _____ inches.

4. The threshold intensity for aerobic fitness improvement is at an exercise heart rate of about _____ percent of maximum.

5. If exercise intensity is below the threshold level of aerobic training, fitness can still improve if exercise _____ is extended.

TRUE / FALSE

_____ 1. The greatest training improvement in max $\dot{V}O_2$ occurs in individuals with the highest initial fitness.

_____ 2. Women who exercise regularly have a noticeably easier time giving birth .

_____ 3. When measuring pulse rate at the carotid artery, avoid pressing too hard because in some people the external pressure can cause the heart rate to speed up.

_____ 4. It is not possible to totally deplete the high energy phosphate pool in specific muscles.

_____ 5. To train the capacity of the anaerobic energy system for a particular sport, any form of exercise can be used as long as it places an overload on anaerobic metabolism.

ACROSS

1 Use of exercise HR enables each person to _____ exercise training
3 This activity is an excellent form of upper body exercise
5 The step test named for a mid-western town
6 A rest-_____ interval is a period of passive recovery in interval training
7 First word abbreviation for RPE
8 Maximum heart rate decreases as a function of _____
9 One way to improve physiological fitness is to increase the _____ of an exercise
12 Fitness improvement is maintained even if this training component is reduced significantly
14 Exercise at or above 50% of one's maxVO2 is necessary to _____ the aerobic system
17 50% of maxVO2 = 70% of this maximum
21 The step-test is a measure of this fitness component
22 A lower recovery heart rate indicates a higher aerobic fitness
24 Blood will tend to do this in peripheral tissues if exercise stops abruptly
25 Initials for professional organization in sports medicine and fitness
26 A muscle that thickens with pressure overload
27 The lower the _____ fitness level, the greater the potential for improvement
28 Rhythmic, big _____ activities are ideal for aerobic exercise training

Chapter 19

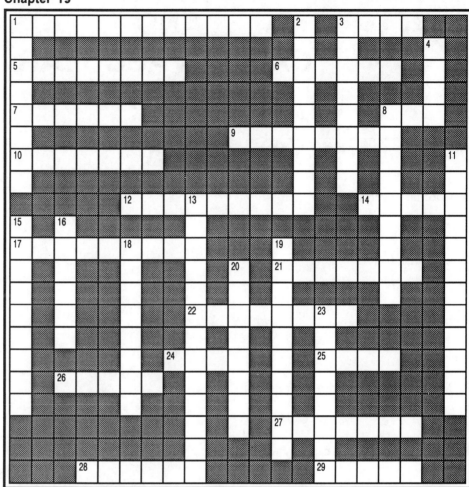

29 One of the _____ of aerobic training is to improve cardiovascular capacity

DOWN

1 This training uses repetitive exercise bouts with specific recovery periods
2 Significant increases in core temperature should be avoided during this period
3 Maximum heart rates are about 13 beats/min lower in this exercise
4 70% of max HR is the threshold for the training sensitive _____
8 High intensity interval training is ideal for conditioning this metabolic system
11 Intensity of training is the most critical factor for successful aerobic _____

13 A step test named for this New York City school
15 70% of max HR is considered a _____ level of cardiovascular stress for aerobic improvement
16 Step test heart rate scores have been used to estimate this criterion for aerobic fitness
18 _____ is prolonged when exercise produces large amounts of lactic acid
19 Repetitive bouts of near-maximum effort produce the highest level of the this anaerobic metabolite
20 The fundamental training principle
23 Successive bouts of heavy exercise interspersed with recovery cause a lactate _____

AGING, EXERCISE, AND CARDIOVASCULAR HEALTH

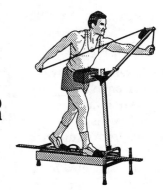

DEFINE KEY TERMS AND CONCEPTS

1. Coronary heart disease

2. CHD risk factors

3. Exercise participation

4. Most prevalent exercise complications

5. Decline in functional capacity with advancing years

6. Maximum strength of men and women

7. Regular physical training facilitates protein retention

8. Joint flexibility

9. Central nervous system function

10. Lung function

11. Decline in aerobic capacity

12. Trainability among older men and women

13. Accumulation of excess fat

14. Improved physical fitness and a vigorous lifestyle may retard the aging process

15. Longevity of former college athletes

16. Harvard alumni

17. Diseases of the heart and blood vessels

18. Coronary circulation

19. Atherosclerosis

20. Ischemic

21. Thrombus

22. Myocardial infarction

23. Angina pectoris

24. Significant heart disease risk factors

25. Primary risk factors

26. Associated risk factors

27. Gender advantage

28. Hyperlipidemia

29. Lipoprotein

30. Hyperlipoproteinemia

31. High-density lipoproteins

32. Low-density lipoproteins

33. Hypertension

34. Systolic hypertension

35. Diastolic hypertension

36. Borderline high blood pressure

37. Cigarette smoking is one of the best predictors of CHD

38. Type A personality

39. Type B personality

40. Risk factors are associated with each other

STUDY QUESTIONS

Participation in physical activity

Describe the average level of exercise participation for the American male and female.

<u>Male</u>

<u>Female</u>

Is exercising safe?

What is the risk of dying suddenly during exercise?

What is the most prevalent form of injury caused by exercise?

Aging and bodily function

Draw a generalized curve that relates the level of body functions to age.

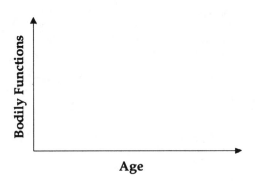

Muscular strength

How much has muscular strength declined by age 70?

Decrease in muscle mass

A reduced muscle mass is a primary factor responsible for what age-associated decrease in physiologic function?

Muscle trainability among the elderly

How much can the elderly increase their strength with a proper resistance training program? (HINT: refer to Figure 20-3 in your textbook.)

Flexibility

Discuss the effects of aging on joint flexibility

Nervous system

What general effect does aging have on the nervous system?

Pulmonary function

How does aging affect pulmonary function?

Cardiovascular function

How does aging affect the cardiovascular system?

What is the maximum heart rate of a person aged 59 years? Show your calculations.

The aerobic system is responsive to training at any age

If middle-aged men train regularly over a 10-year period, what effects will be noted on the following:

Blood pressure

Body mass

Aerobic fitness

Body mass and body fat

How much weight will the average 20-year old male gain by age 60?

Regular exercise: a fountain of youth

List five health benefits of regular physical activity.

     1.

     2.

     3.

     4.

     5.

Discuss whether exercise improves and extends life.

Enhanced quality to a longer life: a study of Harvard alumni

Describe the major findings of the study of Harvard alumni.

Epidemiologic evidence

How does physical <u>inactivity</u> relate to the risk of coronary heart disease?

Improved fitness: a little goes a long way

Explain the major findings of the experiment described in Figure 20-6 of your textbook.

Coronary heart disease

What percentage of total deaths is caused by diseases of the heart and blood vessels?

What is the current economic impact of heart-related diseases?

The heart's blood supply

List the major components of the heart's circulatory network.

A life-long process

At what age can fatty streaks develop in the coronary arteries?

Changes on the cellular level

List three cellular changes that take place in the process of atherosclerosis.

1.

2.

3.

Risk factors for coronary heart disease

List 10 heart disease risk factors.

1.	6.
2.	7.
3.	8.
4.	9.
5.	10.

List three CHD risk factors that are predetermined and cannot be controlled or remedied, and three treatable risk factors.

Predetermined factors	Treatable factors
1.	1.
2.	2.
3.	3.

Age, gender, and heredity

At what age do the chances of dying from CHD increase progressively and dramatically for men and for women? (HINT: refer to Figure 20-10 in your textbook.)

<u>Men</u>   <u>Women</u>

Cholesterol and triglycerides

What are the current standards for desirable levels of total cholesterol and levels above which adults should receive treatment? (HINT: refer to Table 20-1 in your textbook.)

<u>Desirable</u>

<u>Treatment required</u>

The forms of cholesterol are also important

List two characteristics of the lipoproteins HDL and LDL.

<u>HDL</u>   <u>LDL</u>

1.

2.

What is important about the ratio of total cholesterol to HDL cholesterol?

Hypertension

What is the lower borderline limit for the classification of high blood pressure?

<u>Systolic</u>

<u>Diastolic</u>

List four severe medical complications that can result from chronic hypertension.

1.

2.

3.

4.

Exercise is effective

In what way does regular exercise training affect high blood pressure?

Cigarette smoking

List three facts about cigarette smoking and the risk of developing CHD.

1.

2.

3.

Obesity

How does obesity contribute as a multiple risk factor for CHD?

Personality and behavior patterns

What are the personality characteristics of individuals who exhibit Type A and Type B behavior patterns?

<u>Type A</u>

<u>Type B</u>

Physical inactivity

List eight benefits of regular exercise in relation to CHD.

1.   5.

2.   6.

3.   7.

4.   8.

Interaction of risk factors

Discuss the interaction among the primary CHD risk factors.

PRACTICE QUIZ

MULTIPLE CHOICE

1. Generally, maximum heart rate can be estimated:
    a. during all-out sprint activities lasting about 30 seconds
    b. as 220 minus a person's age in years
    c. as 240 minus a person's age in years
    d. only during aerobic exercise
    e. only during anaerobic exercise

2. Generally, after age 30:
    a. there is no change in maximum oxygen uptake
    b. there is no change in nerve conduction velocity
    c. there is a general decline in the body's various functional capacities
    d. brain cells decrease by 10% per year
    e. muscle strength stays about the same

3. The leading cause of death in the U.S. is:
    a. diabetes
    b. pneumonia and influenza
    c. cancer
    d. car accidents
    e. diseases of the heart and blood vessels

4. Name of the crown-like network of arterial vessels that originate at top of the heart:
    a. right ascending artery
    b. right circumflex artery
    c. left circumflex artery
    d. left descending vessel and aorta
    e. coronary circulation

5. A clot that plugs one of the coronary vessels causing a portion of the heart muscle to die is called:
    a. myocardial bolus
    b. myocardial infarction
    c. myocardial fibrillation
    d. myocardial pectoris
    e. myocardial relapse

FILL-IN

1. If your professor is 50 years old, a good estimate of his/her maximum heart rate is _____ beats/min.

2. A study of 17,000 Harvard alumni who entered college between 1916 and 1950 indicated that men who expended about _____ kcal per week in exercise had one-fourth to one-third lower death rates than normal.

3. Death from _____ is the number one killer of women according to the American Heart Association.

4. The heart muscle's elaborate crown-like circulatory network is called the _____ .

5. The chemical modification of compounds like the cholesterol in LDL initiates a complex process that causes bulging lesions in the walls of the coronary arteries. These changes are the first signs of _____.

TRUE / FALSE

_____ 1. The elderly represent the fastest growing segment of the American population, with the average life expectancy for men and women rapidly approaching 80 years.

_____ 2. According to the latest data on the physical activity of non-institutionalized adults aged 18 years and older, only about 44 % of men and 47% of women reported that they engaged in regular vigorous exercise.

_____ 3. Regular exercise decreases CHD risk even if it is only moderate in intensity.

_____ 4. Approximately 80% of the total deaths in the U.S. are caused by diseases of the heart and blood vessels.

_____ 5. Four treatable CHD risk factors are hypertension, physical inactivity, elevated lipids, and smoking.

Chapter 20

ACROSS

5 Degenerative process causing coronary artery narrowing

6 Initials for the most prevalent killer of men and women

7 A group of Harvard _____ was studied to evaluate factors related to CHD and longevity

9 The use of the _____ is the greatest preventable CHD risk

11 Hypertension, cigarette smoking, physical inactivity, and high cholesterol are the four _____ risks for CHD

15 While regular exercise may improve health and well-being, it may have little effect on _____

17 Personality type that may be at risk for heart disease

19 To reduce blood pressure, regular exercise may be most effective for people who are moderately _____

21 This gender group tends to have heart disease later in life

23 This component of blood pressure should not exceed 140 mmHg

25 A _____ of total cholesterol to HDL cholesterol greater than 4.5 is a high CHD risk

26 Regular exercise throughout life can generally override the deterioration in _____ function with age

27 A two word term for factors that increase one's chances of developing heart disease

DOWN

1 At any age, active adults have lower levels of body _____ than less active counterparts

2 A CHD risk factor that cannot be modified

3 _____ flexibility declines 20 to 30% from 30 to 80 years of age

4 Initials for the lipoprotein containing the least amount of cholesterol

6 Component of circulatory system that supplies blood to the heart

8 A protein that transports cholesterol in the blood

9 A two word term to describe individuals who are at greater than normal risk for CHD

10 Diseases of the cardiovascular _____ are the leading cause of death among adults

12 The actual blockage of a coronary vessel

13 Pain caused by inadequate oxygen supply to the myocardium

14 This group (gender) dies younger

16 A word indicating inadequate oxygen supply

17 Thought to be CHD resistant personality

18 Popular term for myocardial infarction

20 Chronic hypertension is often called the "_____" killer

21 For ages 55 to 65, about 6 of every 100 _____ die from CHD

22 Abbreviation for a cardiovascular variable that decreases with age

24 Initials for the lipoprotein that increases with cigarette smoking

SECTION II

• SELF-ASSESSMENT TESTS

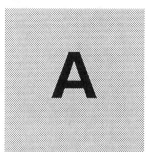

A EATING SMART ASSESSMENT

(Source: American Cancer Society, Rev. 1989, pp. 2-5)

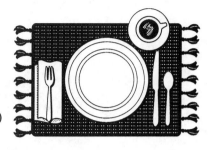

Let's see how "smart" you are in terms of the quality of your food intake. Complete the Eating Smart Assessment and get a broad view of the diversity of your diet, especially its content of fat- and fiber-rich foods. A high rating means that you're on the right track in terms of prudent nutrition to help protect against heart disease and certain cancers.

OILS AND FATS: butter, margarine, shortening, mayonnaise, sour cream, lard, oil	POINTS
I always add these to foods in cooking and/or at the table	____ 0
I occasionally add these to foods in cooking and/or at the table	____ 1
I rarely add these to foods in cooking and/or at the table	____ 2

DAIRY PRODUCTS: milk, yogurt, cheese, ice cream	POINTS
I drink whole milk	____ 0
I drink 1 or 2% fat-free milk	____ 1
I seldom eat frozen desserts or ice cream	____ 2
I eat ice cream almost every day	____ 0
Instead of ice cream, I eat ice milk, low-fat frozen yogurt and sherbet	____ 1
I eat only fruit ices, seldom eat frozen dairy desserts	____ 2
I eat mostly high-fat cheese (jack, cheddar, colby, Swiss, cream)	____ 0
I eat both low- and high-fat cheeses	____ 1
I eat mostly low-fat cheeses (2% cottage, skim milk, mozzarella)	____ 2

SNACKS: potato/corn chips, nuts, buttered popcorn, candy bars	POINTS
I eat these every day	____ 0
I eat some of these occasionally	____ 1
I seldom or never eat these snacks	____ 2

BAKED GOODS : pies, cakes, cookies, sweet rolls, doughnuts	POINTS
I eat them 5 or more times a week	____ 0
I eat them 2-4 times a week	____ 1
I seldom eat baked goods or eat only low-fat baked goods	____ 2

POULTRY AND FISH : (If you do not eat meat, fish, or poultry, give yourself 2 points)	POINTS
I rarely eat these foods	____ 0
I eat them 1-2 times a week	____ 1
I eat them 3 or more times a week	____ 2

LOW-FAT MEATS : extra lean hamburger, round steak, pork loin, roast, tenderloin, chuck roast. (If you do not eat meat, fish, or poultry, give yourself 2 points)	POINTS
I rarely eat these foods	____ 0
I occasionally eat these foods	____ 1
I eat mostly fat-trimmed red meats	____ 2

HIGH-FAT MEATS : luncheon meats, bacon, hot dogs, sausage, steak, regular and lean ground beef. (If youdo not eat meat, fish, or poultry, give yourself 2 points)	POINTS
I eat these every day	____ 0
I occasionally eat these foods	____ 1
I rarely eat these foods	____ 2

CURED AND SMOKED MEAT AND FISH : luncheon meats, hot dogs, bacon, ham and other smoked or pickled meats and fish. (If you do not eat meat, fish, or poultry, give yourself 2 points)	POINTS
I eat these foods 4 or more times a week	____ 0
I eat some of these foods 1-3 times a week	____ 1
I seldom eat these foods	____ 2

LEGUMES : dried beans, peas (kidney, navy, lima, pinto, garbanzo, spit-pea, lentil)	POINTS
I eat legumes less than once a week	____ 0
I eat legumes 1-2 times a week	____ 1
I eat legumes 3 or more times a week	____ 2

WHOLE GRAINS AND CEREALS : whole grain breads, brown rice, pasta, whole grain cereals	POINTS
I seldom eat these foods	____ 0
I eat these foods 1-2 times a day	____ 1
I eat these foods 4 or more times daily	____ 2

VITAMIN-C RICH FRUITS AND VEGETABLES: citrus fruits, juices, green peppers, berries	POINTS
I seldom eat these foods	____ 0
I eat these foods 3-5 times a week	____ 1
I eat these foods 1-2 times a day	____ 2

DARK GREEN AND DEEP YELLOW FRUITS AND VEGETABLES: broccoli, greens, carrots, peaches (dark green and yellow fruits and vegetables contain beta carotene that your body turns into vitamin A. Vitamin A helps protect against certain types of cancer-causing substances)	POINTS
I seldom eat these foods	____ 0
I eat these foods 1-2 times a week	____ 1
I eat these foods 3-4 times a week	____ 2

VEGETABLES OF THE CABBAGE FAMILY: broccoli, cabbage, brussels sprouts, cauliflower	POINTS
I seldom eat these foods	____ 0
I eat these foods 1-2 times a week	____ 1
I eat these foods 3-4 times a week	____ 2

ALCOHOL	POINTS
I drink more than 2 oz daily	____ 0
I drink every week, but not daily	____ 1
I occasionally or never drink alcohol	____ 2

YOUR BODY WEIGHT	POINTS
I am more than 20 lbs over my ideal weight	____ 0
I am 10-20 lbs over my ideal weight	____ 1
I am within 10 lbs of my ideal weight	____ 2

ADD UP YOUR TOTAL POINTS HERE _____

TOTAL POINTS

YOUR EATING SMART RATING

0 - 12 POINTS: A WARNING SIGNAL
Your diet is too high in fat and too low in fiber-rich foods. Assess your eating habits to see where you could make improvements.
13 -1 7 POINTS: NOT BAD
You still have a way to go. Review your quiz to identify those areas in which you rate poorly; then make the necessary adjustments
18 - 36 POINTS: GOOD FOR YOU, YOU'RE EATING SMART
You should feel very good about yourself. You have been careful to limit your fats and eat a varied diet. Keep up the good habits and continue to look for ways to improve.

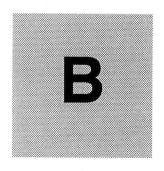

ASSESSMENT OF ENERGY AND NUTRIENT INTAKE

YOUR THREE-DAY DIETARY SURVEY

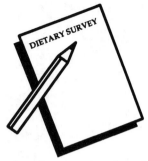

Your three-day dietary survey is a relatively simple yet accurate method to determine the nutritional quality and total calories consumed each day. The secret is to keep a daily log of food intake for any three days that represent your normal eating pattern.

Many experiments have shown that people can accurately calculate caloric intake from records of their daily food consumption that are usually within 10% of the number of calories actually consumed. For example, suppose the caloric value of your daily food intake was directly measured in the bomb calorimeter and averaged 2130 kcal. If you kept a three-day dietary history and estimated your caloric intake, the daily value would likely be within 10% of the actual value, or between 1920 kcal and 2350 kcal. As long as you maintained a careful record, the degree of accuracy for daily determinations would be within acceptable limits.

Before recording your daily caloric intake over the three-day period, you should become familiar with "honest" calorie counting. This requires four items for measuring food: a plastic ruler, a standard measuring cup, measuring spoons, and an inexpensive balance or weighing scale. You can purchase these items at most hardware stores. Second, familiarize yourself with the nutritional and caloric values of foods by consulting food labels and Appendix D in your textbook. Listed under "specialty and fast-food items" at the end of the Appendix are the nutritional values for food items sold at fast-food chain stores. You also can obtain an inexpensive calorie-counting guide at newsstands and bookstores that gives the nutrient and energy values for most foods. Guides that list foods according to brand names are also helpful .

Measure or weigh each of the food items in your diet. This is the only reliable way to obtain an accurate estimate of the size of a food portion. If you elect to use Appendix D in the text to estimate the nutritional and kcal values, you only need to weigh each food item. If you use a supplementary calorie-counting guide, this may require the measuring cup, spoons, and ruler.

Food Categories

Meat and Fish

Measure the portion of meat or fish by thickness, length, and width, or record weight on the scale.

Vegetables, Mashed Potatoes, Rice, Cereals, Salads

Measure the portion in a measuring cup or record weight on the scale.

Cream or Sugar Added to Coffee or Tea

Measure the portion with the measuring spoons before adding to the drink or record weight on the scale.

Fluids and Bottled Drinks

Check the labels for volume or empty the container into the measuring cup. If you weigh the fluid, be sure to subtract the weight of the cup or glass. Sugar-free soft drinks usually have kcal values listed on their labels.

Cookies, Cakes, Pies

For these items, measure the diameter and thickness with a ruler, or weigh on the scale. Evaluate frosting or sauces separately.

Fruits

Cut them in half before eating and measure the diameters, or weigh them on the scale. For fruits that must be peeled or have rinds or cores, be sure the weight of the non-edible portion is subtracted from the total weight of the food. Do this for items such as oranges, apples, and bananas.

Jam, Salad Dressing, Catsup, Mayonnaise

Measure the condiment with the measuring spoon or weigh the portion on the scale.

Directions For Computing Your Three-Day Dietary Survey

Step 1. Prepare a table (similar to Table B-1) indicating the intake of food items during a day. Include the amount (g or oz), caloric value, and for carbohydrate, fat, and protein content as well as the minerals Ca^{++} and Fe^{++}, and vitamins C, B_1 (thiamine), and B_2 (riboflavin), total fiber , and cholesterol. The Tables for specialty and fast-food items in Appendix D do not contain information about fiber and cholesterol content. However, these data can be "guesstimated" by relating a particular fast-food item to a similar one in the main portion of the Appendix.

Step 2. Be sure to list <u>each</u> food you consume for breakfast, lunch, and dinner, and between meal eating, and snacks. Include food items that are used in preparing the meal (e.g., butter, oils, margarine, bread crumbs, egg coating, etc.).

Step 3. Weigh, measure, or approximate the size of each portion of food that you eat. Record these values on your daily record chart (e.g., 3 oz of salad oil, 1/8 piece of 8" diameter apple pie, etc.).

Step 4. Record your daily calorie and nutrient intake on a chart similar to Table B-1 for a 21- year old college student. Record the daily totals for the caloric and nutrient headings on the "Daily and Average Daily Summary Chart" (Table B-2). When you've completed your three-day survey, compute the three-day total by adding up the values for days 1, 2, and 3 and divide by 3 to determine the daily average of each nutrient category.

Step 5. Using each of the average daily nutrient values, calculate the percent of the RDA consumed for that

Step 6. Remember to be as accurate and honest as possible. <u>Do not</u> include unusual or atypical days in your dietary survey (e.g., days that you are sick, special occasions such as birthdays, or eating out at restaurants unless that is normal for you).

Step 7. Remember that the protein RDA is equal to 0.8 g protein per kilogram of body weight (1 kg = 2.2 lbs).

Step 8. Compute the percent of your total calories supplied from carbohydrate, fat, and protein.

> For example, if total average daily caloric intake is 2450 kcal/day, and 1600 kcal are from carbohydrates, the daily percent of total calories from carbohydrates is:
> 1600/2450 X 100 = 65%

Step 9. While there is no specific RDA for fat or carbohydrate, a prudent recommendation is that fat should not exceed more than 30% of your total caloric intake; for active men and women, carbohydrates should be approximately 60% of the total calories ingested. Thus, in computing the percent of RDA for graphing purposes in Figure B-1 you should assume that:

> a. RDA for fat as 30% of total calories
> b. RDA for carbohydrate as 60% of total calories

> For example, if 50% of your average daily calories comes from fat, you are taking in 167% of the recommended value (RDA) for this nutrient: [50% divided by 30% (recommended percentage) X 100 =167%]

Step 10. As was the case for fat and carbohydrate, there is no RDA for daily caloric intake. Any recommendation for energy intake needs to be based on one's present status for body fat as well as current daily energy expenditure. However, average values for daily caloric intake have been published for the typical young adult and equal about 2100 kcal for young women and 3000 kcal for young men. Thus, for graphing purposes in Figure B-1 you can evaluate your average daily caloric intake against the "average" values for your gender and age.

> For example, if you are a 20-year old female and you consume an average of 2400 kcal daily, your energy intake would be equal to 114% of the average (RDA) for your age and gender: [2400 kcal divided by 2100 kcal (average) X 100 = 114%]. This does not mean that you need to go on a diet and reduce food intake to bring you in line with the average U.S. value. On the contrary, your higher than average caloric intake may be required to power your active lifestyle that contributes to maintaining a desirable body mass and body composition.

If you eat a food item not listed in Appendix D or in a calorie guide, try to make an intelligent guess as to its composition and the amount you have eaten. It is better to overestimate the amount of food consumed than to underestimate or to make no estimation at all. If you go to a restaurant for dinner, or to a friend's house where it may be inappropriate to measure the food, then omit this day from the counting procedure and resume record keeping the following day.

Because the purpose of keeping records for three days is to obtain an accurate appraisal for the average daily energy and nutrient intake, record-keeping is extremely important. **Be sure to record everything you eat.** If you are not completely "honest" you are wasting your time. Most people find it easier to keep accurate records if they record food items while preparing a meal or immediately afterwards when eating snack items.

Table B-1. Sample one-day caloric and nutrient intake for a 21-year old college student.

Food Item	Amount	kcal	Protein g	CHO g	Fat g	Ca^{++} mg	Fe^{++} mg	Fiber g	Cholesterol mg	Thiam* mg	Ribofl* mg
Breakfast											
eggs, hard boiled	2 (2oz ea)	160	14.1	1.4	11.2	55.2	1.9	0.0	452	0.06	0.53
orange juice	8 oz	104	0.9	86.4	0.5	72.4	0.8	0.9	0.0	0.20	0.06
corn flakes	1 cup/1 oz	110	2.3	24.4	0.5	1.0	1.8	0.6	0.0	0.37	0.42
skim milk	8 oz	80	7.8	10.6	0.6	279.2	0.1	0.0	3.7	0.08	0.32
Snack											
none											
Lunch											
tuna fish (oil pack)	2 oz	112	16.5	0.0	68.0	7.8	0.8	0.0	10.0	0.02	0.06
white bread (toast)	2 pieces	168	5.3	31.4	2.5	81.2	1.8	1.3	0.0	0.24	0.21
mayonnaise	1 oz	203	0.3	0.8	22.6	5.7	0.2	0.0	16.8	0.01	0.01
skim milk	8 oz	80	7.8	10.6	0.6	279.2	0.1	0.0	3.7	0.08	0.32
plums	4 (2 oz ea)	128	1.8	29.5	1.4	10.3	0.2	4.4	0.0	0.10	0.22
Snack											
chocolate milkshake	8oz	288	7.7	46.4	8.4	256	0.7	0.3	29.6	0.13	0.55
Dinner											
sirloin steak, lean	8 oz	456	64.8	0.0	20.2	18.6	5.8	0.0	173.6	0.21	0.47
french fries, veg oil	6 oz	540	6.8	67.2	28.1	34.2	1.3	3.4	0.0	0.30	0.05
cole slaw	4 oz	80	1.4	14.1	3.0	51.2	0.7	2.3	9.2	0.08	0.07
Italian bread	2 oz	156	5.1	32.0	1.0	9.4	1.5	0.9	0.0	0.23	0.13
light beer	8 oz	96	0.6	8.8	0.0	11.2	0.1	0.5	0.0	0.02	0.06
Snack											
yogurt whole milk	6 oz	102	5.9	7.9	5.5	205.8	0.1	0.0	22.1	0.05	0.24
Daily Total		2863	149.1	371.5	174.1	1378.4	17.2	14.6	720.7	2.18	3.72

* Thiam = Thiamine; Ribofl = Riboflavin

Table B-2. Daily and Average Daily Summary chart of the intake of calories and specific food nutrients

Day	kcal	Protein* g	Lipid* g	CHO* g	Ca++ mg	Fe++ mg	Thiamine mg	Riboflavin mg	Fiber g	Cholesterol mg
#1										
#2										
#3										
Three day total										
Average Daily Value**										

* Use the following calorific transformations to convert your average daily grams of carbohydrate (CHO), lipid, and protein to average daily calories:

1 g CHO	=	4 kcal
1 g Lipid	=	9 kcal
1 g Protein	=	4 kcal

** The Average Daily Value is used to determine the percent of the RDA for your graph. See Table B-2 for sample calculations. Figure B-1 is a bar graph showing the nutrient values as a percent of the average or recommended value for each item.

ASSESSMENT OF ENERGY AND NUTRIENT INTAKE

Table B-3. RDA values for selected nutrients including sample computations for deriving the percent of RDA from your dietary survey. Each of the values listed in the table are 100% values for purposes of graphing your dietary survey. Recommended Dietary Allowances, Revised - 1989. [Source: Food and Nutrition Board, National Academy of Sciences , National Research Council, Washington, D.C.]

MEN

Age	kcal*	Protein g/kg	Ca^{++} mg	Fe^{++} mg	Thiamine mg	Riboflavin mg	Fiber* g	Cholesterol* mg
19-22	3000	0.8	1200	10	1.5	1.7	30	300
23-50	2700	0.8	800	10	1.5	1.7	30	300

WOMEN

Age	kcal*	Protein g/kg	Ca^{++} mg	Fe^{++} mg	Thiamine mg	Riboflavin mg	Fiber* g	Cholesterol* mg
19-22	2100	0.8	1200	15	1.1	1.3	30	300
23-50	2000	0.8	800	15	1.1	1.3	30	300

*There is no RDA for daily caloric intake or for the intake of fiber or cholesterol. Value for caloric intake represents an average for adult Americans while fiber and cholesterol values are recommended as being prudent for maintaining good health.

How To Determine The Percentage Of The RDA From Your Dietary Survey

Example #1: Percentage of RDA for protein for a 70-kg person

Daily Protein Intake = 68 g
RDA = (70 kg X 0.8 g/kg) = 56 g
% of RDA = 56 / 68 X 100 = 121%

Example #2: Percentage of RDA for iron (female)

Daily iron intake = 7.5 mg
RDA = 15 mg
% of RDA = 7.5 / 15 X 100 = 50%

Figure B-1. Example of bar graph to illustrate food and nutrient intake as percentage of recommended values.

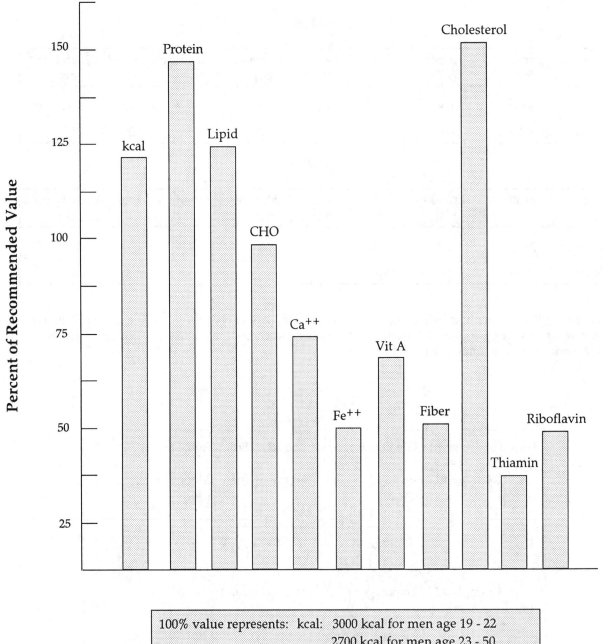

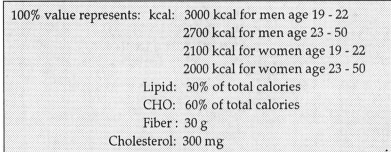

100% value represents: kcal: 3000 kcal for men age 19 - 22
2700 kcal for men age 23 - 50
2100 kcal for women age 19 - 22
2000 kcal for women age 23 - 50
Lipid: 30% of total calories
CHO: 60% of total calories
Fiber : 30 g
Cholesterol: 300 mg

ASSESSMENT OF ENERGY AND NUTRIENT INTAKE

C

ASSESSMENT OF PHYSICAL ACTIVITY
YOUR THREE-DAY ACTIVITY RECALL

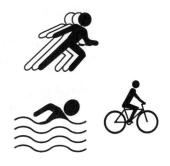

Any hope of changing the pattern and quantity of daily physical activity must be predicated on an accurate appraisal of the daily energy expenditure.

STEP 1. Determine your daily pattern of physical activity, including such minimal daily requirements as sleeping, eating, sitting in class, and bathing. An activity profile can be constructed by keeping a <u>daily log</u> for three days of the actual time allotted to the various activities that represent your usual pattern of activity. To illustrate the procedure, Table C-1 shows a fairly detailed activity profile for a college professor during a typical day of summer vacation. This record includes a description of the activity, its duration, and the calories expended during the activity. For this professor, if it were not for the hour and a half devoted to his daily run, his total daily energy expenditure would be just slightly above average.

STEP 2 (a) Determine your Basal Metabolic Rate (BMR) in kcal/min as follows:

> **MEN:** BMR (kcal/hr) = 38 kcal/m^2/hr* X surface area (m^2)**
>
> **WOMEN:** BMR (kcal/hr) = 35 kcal/m^2/hr* X surface area (m^2)**

* For added precision, determine BMR (kcal/m^2/hr) for your specific age and gender from Figure 13-7 in your textbook.
** Surface area (m^2) is determined from stature and body mass in Figure 13-8 in your textbook.

(b) Divide the BMR value in kcal/hr obtained in Step 2(a) by 60 to compute the BMR value per minute. This value will be used to represent your energy expenditure per minute during sleep.

> **EXAMPLE OF BMR CALCULATIONS**
> *DATA: MALE*
> Age, 40 y
> Stature, 182 cm (72 in)
> Body mass, 86.4 kg (190 lb)
> Body surface area (from Fig. 13-8) = 2.09 m^2
> *CALCULATIONS*
> a. kcal/m^2/hr (from Fig. 13-6) = 37.2
> b. kcal/hr = 37.2 X 2.09 = 77.7
> c. kcal/min = 77.7 / 60 = 1.3

STEP 3. Determine the energy expenditure in kcal/min for each of the activities listed in your profile (For sleep use the BMR computed in Step 2). These values are listed in Appendix A of your textbook. The values **are gross values** that include the resting energy value. If an activity is not included in Appendix A, choose an activity most similar to the one on your list.

STEP 4. Multiply the tabled energy expenditure values by the number of minutes spent in each activity.

STEP 5. Sum the total energy expenditure for each activity, including the value for sleep, to arrive at your <u>total</u> energy expenditure for the day.

STEP 6. Repeat steps 2-5 for each of the three days. Obtain the average daily energy expenditure for the three day period by summing the total calories expended over the three day period, and divide by 3.

HOW TO INTERPRET YOUR AVERAGE DAILY ENERGY EXPENDITURE

There is no norm or desirable standard for the number of calories you should expend during a day. Many factors, including body size, age, gender, and most importantly, level of physical activity are involved. The average daily energy expenditure is 3000 kcal for men and 2100 kcal for women between the ages of 19 and 22 years. If you are not gaining or losing body mass, then your energy expenditure equal s your energy intake.

Table C-1. Detailed record of physical activity for one day for a university professor

Activity	Begin Time	End Time	Total Minutes	Similar Activity Appendix A	kcal/min	Total kcal
wake, bathroom use	6:45AM	6:53	8	standing quietly	2.3	18.4
go back to bed	6:53	7:30	38	BMR	1.3	48.1
eat breakfast	7:30	7:50	10	eating, sitting	2.0	40.0
use bathroom	7:50	8:00	10	standing quietly	2.3	23.0
dress	8:00	8:06	6	standing quietly	2.3	13.8
drive to school	8:06	8:17	11	sitting quietly	2.0	22.0
walk to office	8:17	8:25	8	walking, normal pace	6.9	55.8
work in office, pick-up mail	8:25	10:00	95	writing, sitting	2.5	237.5
up/down stairs	10:00	10:10	10	11 min 30 sec pace	11.7	117.0
work in office	10:10	12:10PM	120	writing, sitting	2.5	300
go to locker	12:10	12:12	2	walking, normal pace	6.9	13.8
get dressed	12:12	12:16	4	standing quietly	2.3	9.2
walk to track	12:16	12:20	4	walk, normal pace	6.9	27.6
wait for friend	12:20	12:30	10	standing quietly	2.3	23.0
run to park, back	12:30	2:00	90	8-min mile pace	17.17	1553
walk to locker	2:00	2:04	4	walk, normal pace	6.9	27.6
shower, dress	2:04	2:20	16	quiet standing	2.3	36.8
walk to office	2:20	2:24	4	walk, normal pace	6.9	27.6
meeting/lunch	2:24	3:00	36	eating, sitting	2.0	72.0
work in office	3:00	5:05	125	writing, sitting	2.5	312.5
walk to library	5:05	5:12	7	walk, normal pace	6.9	48.3
work in library	5:12	6:05	53	writing, sitting	2.5	132.5
walk to dean	6.05	6:10	5	walk, normal pace	6.9	34.5
meeting, dean	6:10	6:35	25	writing sitting	2.5	62.5
walk to office	6:35	6:43	8	walk, normal pace	6.9	55.2
walk to car	6:43	6:51	8	walk, normal pace	6.9	55.2
drive home	6:51	7:03	12	sitting quietly	1.8	21.6
change clothes	7:03	7:07	4	standing quietly	2.3	9.2
wash-up	7:07	7:11	4	standing quietly	2.3	9.2
cook dinner	7:11	8:00	49	cooking	4.1	200.9
watch TV	8:00	8:30	30	sitting quietly	1.8	54.0
eat dinner	8:30	9:00	30	eating, sitting	2.0	60.0
mail letter	9:00	9:05	5	walk, normal pace	6.9	34.5
listen to stereo	9:05	9:30	25	sitting quietly	1.8	45.0
watch TV	9:30	10:30	60	sitting quietly	1.8	108
wash-up	10:30	10:38	8	standing quietly	2.3	18.4
read in bed	10:38	11:15	37	lying at ease	1.9	70.3
turn off lights	11:15	6:15AM	450	BMR	1.3	585.0

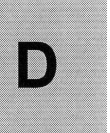

ASSESSMENT OF EXERCISE READINESS (PAR-Q)

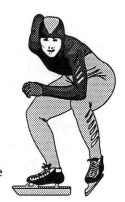

To get a general idea of whether you are physically ready to exercise, complete the following Physical Activity Readiness Questionnaire (The PAR-Q*).

PAR-Q is designed to help you help yourself. Many health benefits are associated with regular exercise, and the completion of PAR-Q is a sensible first step if you are planning to increase your physical activity. For most people, physical activity should not pose any problem or hazard. PAR-Q has been designed to identify the small number of adults for whom physical activity might be inappropriate or those who should have medical advice concerning the type of activity most suitable for them.

> **COMMON SENSE IS YOUR BEST GUIDE IN ANSWERING THESE QUESTIONS. PLEASE READ EACH QUESTION CAREFULLY AND CHECK *YES* OR *NO* IF IT APPLIES TO YOU.**

YES _____ NO _____ 1. Has your doctor ever said you have heart trouble?

YES _____ NO _____ 2. Do you frequently have pains in your heart and chest?

YES _____ NO _____ 3. Do you often feel faint or have spells of severe dizziness?

YES _____ NO _____ 4. Has a doctor ever said your blood pressure was too high?

YES _____ NO _____ 5. Has your doctor told you that you have a bone or joint problem that has been aggravated by exercise, or might be made worse with exercise?

YES _____ NO _____ 6. Is there a good physical reason not mentioned here why you should not follow an activity program even if you wanted to?

YES _____ NO _____ 7. Are you over age 65 and not accustomed to vigorous exercise?

*PAR-Q was developed by the British Columbia Ministry of Health. Conceptualized and critiqued by the Multidisciplinary Advisory Board on Exercise (MABE). Reference: PAR-Q Validation Report, British Columbia Ministry of Health, May, 1978.

IF YOU ANSWERED *YES* TO ONE OR MORE OF THE QUESTIONS

If you have not recently done so, consult with your personal physician by telephone or in person **BEFORE** increasing your physical activity and/or taking a fitness test. Show your doctor a copy of this quiz. After medical evaluation, seek advice from your physician as to your suitability for :

- Unrestricted physical activity, probably on a gradually increasing basis.
- Restricted or supervised activity to meet your specific needs, at least on an initial basis. Check in your community for special programs or services.

IF YOU ANSWERED *NO* TO ALL OF THE QUESTIONS

If you answered PAR-Q accurately, you have reasonable assurance of your present suitability for:

- *A graduated exercise program* - a gradual increase in proper exercise promotes good fitness development while minimizing or eliminating discomfort.
- *An exercise test* - simple tests of fitness (such as the Canadian Home Fitness Test) or more complex types may be undertaken if you so desire.
- *Postpone exercising* - if you have a temporary minor illness, such as a common cold, postpone any exercise program.

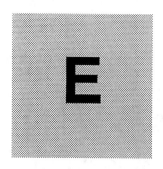

E

ASSESSMENT OF HEALTH- RELATED PHYSICAL FITNESS

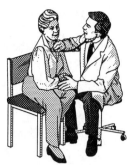

The trend in fitness assessment over the past 20 years has been to deemphasize physical fitness tests that stress motor performance and athletic fitness (i.e., tests of speed, power, balance, and agility). The modern trend is to focus on those measures of fitness that assess functional capacity and also reflect various aspects of overall good health or disease prevention, or both. The four components of health-related physical fitness that are commonly evaluated include aerobic power (cardiorespiratory fitness), body composition, abdominal muscular strength and endurance, and lower back and hamstring flexibility. An upper extremity measure of muscular strength is also often included in the fitness profile although it is not related to health status in a direct way.

A person's performance on each of the test items of health-related fitness is not fixed; rather, tests of health-related fitness can be significantly improved through a program of regular exercise and weight control.

TEST COMPONENT #1 - LOWER BACK FLEXIBILITY

A. Rationale

A substantial amount of clinical evidence indicates that maintenance of trunk, hip, lower back, and posterior thigh flexibility is important in the prevention and alleviation of lower back pain and tension. Back disorders are associated with weak muscles in the abdominal area and limited range of motion of the lower spine. There is also reduced elasticity of the hamstring muscles at the back of the upper leg. The importance of lower back flexibility as a health-related fitness measure is further supported by the fact that physicians frequently prescribe specific trunk and thigh flexibility stretches for their patients with lower back problems, or for individuals who desire to prevent the occurrence of such problems.

B. Lower Back Flexibility Assessment Test: The Sit and Reach Test

Sit on a mat with your legs extended. Your feet should rest against the base of a plywood box on which a yardstick is mounted with the 9 inch (23 cm) mark on the near side of the box (see Figure E-1). After a general warm-up that includes stretching of the lower back and posterior thighs, slowly reach forward with both hands as far as possible and hold the position momentarily. Record the distance reached on the yardstick by your fingertips. Use the best of four trials as your flexibility score.

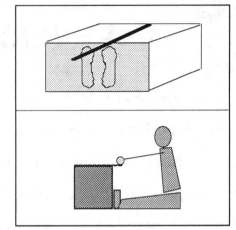

Figure E-1. Sit and reach flexibility test.

C. How Do You Rate on Lower Back Flexibility?

Compare your results with the normative data in Table E-1.

Table E-1. Norms for the sit and reach (cm) for young adult men and women, age 18-21 yr.

Percentile	Men				Women			
	18	19	20	21	18	19	20	21
99	50	49	49	50	52	52	51	50
95	45	45	46	45	47	47	46	46
90	42	43	43	42	46	45	45	44
85	41	42	41	41	44	43	43	43
80	40	40	41	40	43	42	42	42
75	39	39	40	39	42	41	41	42
70	38	38	39	38	40	41	39	40
65	37	37	38	36	40	40	38	39
60	36	36	37	35	39	38	38	38
55	35	35	36	35	38	38	37	37
50	34	34	35	33	38	37	37	36
45	34	33	34	32	37	36	36	36
40	32	32	33	31	36	36	35	35
35	31	31	32	31	35	34	34	34
30	30	29	31	30	34	33	33	33
25	29	28	30	28	33	32	32	32
20	27	27	27	27	32	31	31	31
15	25	26	25	25	30	29	30	29
10	23	23	22	24	29	27	28	27
5	19	19	18	20	26	23	24	25

From: American Alliance For Health, Physical Education, Recreation, and Dance: Norms For College Students: Health Related Physical Fitness Test. Reston, VA, 1985.

TEST COMPONENT #2 - PERCENT BODY FAT

A. Rationale

Body composition is defined as the relative percentage of fat and fat-free body mass. An excessive accumulation of body fat significantly hinders the ability to perform tasks requiring speed, endurance, and coordination. Additionally, research indicates that an excess amount of body fat is an associative and/or contributing factor to four categories of health hazards: (1) disturbance of normal body functions; (2) increased risk of disease (e.g., hypertension, diabetes, coronary heart disease); (3) exacerbation of existing disease states; and (4) adverse physiological effects.

B. Percent Body Fat Assessment Test; Measurement of Fatfolds

Evaluation of body fat can be made by different indirect procedures. These can include *girths* or *fatfolds* measured at specific body sites. In the text we described how to use girth measurements to estimate percent body fat. In this section we describe the alternative method using fatfolds. The fatfold measurements are:

> **MEN: Chest, Abdomen, Thigh**
>
> **WOMEN: Triceps, Suprailium, Thigh**

Measurements at each site are taken in accordance with standard procedures. The exact anatomical sites for each fatfold measurement are described in your textbook in Chapter 14.

> **Abdomen** *(Men only):* Vertical fold measured 1 inch to the right of the umbilicus.
>
> **Chest** *(Men only):* A diagonal fold taken one-half of the distance between the anterior axillary line and the nipple.
>
> **Suprailium** *(Women only):* Slightly oblique fold just above the crest of the hip bone. The fold is lifted to follow the natural diagonal line at this point.
>
> **Thigh** *(Men and Women):* Vertical fold measured at the anterior midline of the thigh, midway between the knee cap and the hip.
>
> **Triceps** *(Women only):* Vertical fold measured at the posterior midline of the upper arm halfway between the tip of the shoulder and the tip of the elbow. The elbow should be extended and relaxed.

Table E-2. Percent fat estimates for **Men**. Sum of chest, abdominal and thigh fatfolds

Sum Fatfolds mm	AGE TO THE LAST YEAR			
	Under 22	23 to 27	28 to 32	33 to 37
8-10	1.3	1.8	2.3	2.9
11-13	2.2	2.8	3.3	3.9
14-16	3.2	3.8	4.3	4.8
17-19	4.2	4.7	5.3	5.8
20-22	5.1	5.7	6.2	6.8
23-25	6.1	6.6	7.2	7.7
26-28	7.0	7.6	8.1	8.7
29-31	8.0	8.5	9.1	9.6
32-34	8.9	9.4	10.0	10.5
35-37	9.8	10.4	10.9	11.5
38-40	10.7	11.3	11.8	12.4
41-43	11.6	12.2	12.7	13.3
44-46	12.0	13.1	13.6	14.2
47-49	13.4	13.9	14.5	15.1
50-52	14.3	14.8	15.4	15.9
53-55	15.1	15.7	16.2	16.8
56-58	16.0	16.5	17.1	17.7
59-61	16.9	17.4	17.9	18.5
62-64	17.6	18.2	18.8	19.4
65-67	18.5	19.0	19.6	20.2
68-70	19.3	19.9	20.4	21.0
71-73	20.1	20.7	21.2	21.8
74-76	20.9	21.5	22.0	22.6
77-79	21.7	22.2	22.8	23.4
80-82	22.4	23.0	23.6	24.2
83-85	23.2	23.8	24.4	25.0
86-88	24.0	24.5	25.1	25.7
89-91	24.7	25.3	25.9	25.5
92-94	25.4	26.0	26.6	27.2
95-97	26.1	26.7	27.3	27.9
98-100	26.9	27.4	28.0	28.6
101-103	27.5	28.1	28.7	29.3
104-106	28.2	28.8	29.4	30.0
107-109	28.9	29.5	30.1	30.7
110-112	29.6	30.2	30.8	31.4
113-115	30.2	30.8	31.4	32.0
116-118	30.9	31.5	32.1	32.7
119-121	31.5	32.1	32.7	33.3
122-124	32.1	32.7	33.3	33.9
125-127	32.7	33.3	33.9	34.9

From: Jackson, A.S. and M.L. Pollock. Practical Assessment of Body Composition. Phys. Sportsmed., 13 (5): 76, 1985 Reproduced with permission of McGraw-Hill Inc.

Table E-3. Percent fat estimates for **Women**. Sum of triceps, suprailium, and thigh fatfolds

Sum Fatfolds mm	AGE TO THE LAST YEAR Under 22	23 to 27	28 to 32	33 to 37
23-25	9.7	9.9	10.2	10.4
26-28	11.0	11.2	11.5	11.7
29-31	12.3	12.5	12.8	13.0
32-34	13.6	13.8	14.0	14.3
35-37	14.8	15.0	15.3	15.5
38-40	16.0	16.3	16.5	16.7
41-43	17.2	17.4	17.7	17.9
44-46	18.3	18.6	18.8	19.1
47-49	19.5	19.7	20.0	20.2
50-52	20.6	20.8	21.1	21.3
53-55	21.7	21.9	22.1	22.4
56-58	22.7	23.0	23.2	23.4
59-61	23.7	24.0	24.2	24.5
62-64	24.7	25.0	25.2	25.5
65-67	25.7	25.9	26.2	26.4
68-70	26.6	26.9	27.1	27.4
71-73	27.5	27.8	28.0	28.3
74-76	28.4	28.7	28.9	29.2
77-79	29.3	29.5	29.8	30.0
80-82	30.1	30.4	30.6	30.9
83-85	30.9	31.2	31.4	31.7
86-88	31.7	32.0	32.2	32.5
89-91	32.5	32.7	33.0	33.2
92-94	33.2	33.4	33.7	33.9
95-97	33.9	34.1	34.4	34.6
98-100	34.6	34.8	35.1	35.3
101-103	35.3	35.4	35.7	35.9
104-106	35.8	36.1	36.3	36.6
107-109	36.4	36.7	36.9	37.1
110-112	37.0	37.2	37.5	37.7
113-115	37.5	37.8	38.0	38.2
116-118	38.0	38.3	38.5	38.8
119-121	38.5	38.7	39.0	39.2
122-124	39.0	39.2	39.4	39.7
125-127	39.4	39.6	39.9	40.1
128-130	39.8	40.0	40.3	40.5

*From: Jackson, A.S., and M.L. Pollock. Practical Assessment of Body Composition. Phys. Sportsmed. 13 (5): 76, 1985. Reproduced with permission of McGraw-Hill Inc.

Compute your percent body fat from the sum of the three fatfold measures as indicated in Table E-2 (men) and Table E-3 (women). Then, see how you rate by determining your percent body fat percentile ranking from the normative standards in Table E-4.

Table E-4. Percentile norms (in percent of fat and percentiles) for the percent body fat test for men and women.*

Percentile	Males	Females
95	6.7	16.8
90	8.1	18.1
85	9.8	19.8
80	10.8	20.8
75	11.6	21.6
70	12.4	22.4
65	13.1	23.1
60	13.7	23.7
55	14.4	24.4
50	15.0	25.0
45	15.6	25.6
40	16.3	26.3
35	16.9	26.9
30	17.6	27.6
25	18.4	28.4
20	19.2	29.2
15	20.2	30.2
10	21.9	31.9

*Normative standards are based on an average body fat for males of 15% and 25% for females with one standard deviation of ± 5% body fat for both genders. McArdle, W.D., et.al.: Exercise Physiology: Energy, Nutrition, and Human Performance. 3rd Edition. Philadelphia: Lea & Febiger, 1991.

TEST COMPONENT #3 - AEROBIC / CARDIOVASCULAR FUNCTION

A. Rationale

Enhanced aerobic-cardiovascular function permits higher levels of extended energy expenditure and physical working capacity, and also facilitates recovery. Also, lack of regular exercise (with a reduced aerobic fitness) has been linked to an increased risk of heart disease.

B. Aerobic - Cardiovascular Assessment Test: The One Mile Run

Aerobic-cardiovascular performance during exercise can be measured by running performance over a distance of one mile. Warm-up for several minutes, then run/walk as rapidly as possible for one mile, and record your time to the nearest second. This test can be performed on a quarter-mile (440 yd) track.

C. How Do You Rate on Aerobic - Cardiovascular Function?

Compare your mile run times with the normative data in Table E-5.

Table E-5. Percentile norms for the mile run (min:sec) for age and gender

Percentile	Men				Women			
	18	19	20	21	18	19	20	21
99	4:57	5:00	4:33	4:38	5:33	5:27	5:16	6:26
95	5:29	5:30	5:21	5:28	7:01	6:56	7:00	7:02
90	5:43	5:42	5:40	5:47	7:28	7:22	7:21	7:21
85	5:55	5:55	5:46	6:01	7:47	7:45	7:41	7:35
80	6:05	6:04	5:59	6:09	8:01	8:00	7:59	7:47
75	6:13	6:09	6:08	6:15	8:15	8:13	8:15	8:01
70	6:21	6:15	6:15	6:22	8:31	8:25	8:30	8:09
65	6:28	6:25	6:23	6:31	8:48	8:34	8:40	8:16
60	6:35	6:32	6:30	6:39	8:59	8:52	8:56	8:30
55	6:40	6:39	6:35	6:47	9:06	9:01	9:07	8:40
50	6:48	6:45	6:43	6:53	9:23	9:13	9:20	8:57
45	6:55	6:53	6:51	6:57	9:35	9:26	9:29	9:04
40	7:03	7:01	6:56	7:02	9:49	9:41	9:43	9:24
35	7:10	7:09	7:09	7:09	10:01	10:00	9:45	9:51
30	7:17	7:15	7:19	7:20	10:16	10:07	10:10	10:02
25	7:29	7:27	7:29	7:34	10:35	10:25	10:28	10:30
20	7:45	7:45	7:41	7:49	10:50	11:00	10:45	11:00
15	8:05	8:00	7:56	8:07	11:17	11:18	11:00	11:20
10	8:33	8:30	8:30	8:29	12:00	12:00	11:30	12:13
5	9:40	9:31	9:48	9:22	13:01	13:05	12:39	12:57

From: American Alliance For Health, Physical Education, Recreation, and Dance: <u>Norms For College Students: Health Related Physical Fitness Test</u>. Reston, VA, 1985.

TEST COMPONENT #4 - ABDOMINAL MUSCULAR STRENGTH AND ENDURANCE

A. Rationale

Abdominal muscular strength and endurance are important in stabilizing the torso while performing diverse physical tasks involving muscular effort. From a health-related fitness perspective, the functional capacity of this muscle group is of considerable importance to the maintenance of proper posture and spinal alignment, and to provide muscular support to reduce lower back strain. Clinical evidence implicates weak muscles of the abdominal wall as a major cause of lower back pain; strengthening these muscles is consistently recommended in both preventive and rehabilitative back programs.

B. Abdominal Muscular Strength and Endurance Assessment: The Modified Sit-Up Test

Lie on your back with knees flexed, feet flat on floor, heels between 12 and 18 inches from the buttocks (see Figure E-2). Cross your arms over your chest with the hands on opposite shoulders. Have your partner hold your feet to keep them in touch with the floor. Curl to the sitting position; arm contact with the chest must be maintained, and the chin should remain tucked to the chest. The sit-up is completed when your elbows touch your thighs. Return to the starting position until your mid-back contacts the floor.

Your partner gives the signal "**Ready, Go.**" The test is started on the word "**Go,**" and ceases on the word "**Stop.**" The number of correctly executed sit-ups performed in 60 seconds is your score. You may rest during the test if necessary.

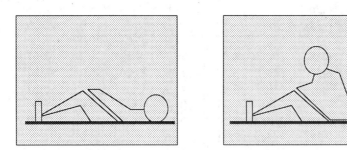

Figure E-2. Example of the modified sit-up

C. *How Do You Rate on Abdominal Muscular Strength and Endurance?*

Compare your abdominal muscular strength and endurance with the normative data in Table E-6.

Table E-6. Percentile norms for one-minute timed sit-ups for age and gender

Percentile	Men				Women			
	18	19	20	21	18	19	20	21
99	70	69	65	67	61	62	63	67
95	62	60	54	61	54	52	53	54
90	57	57	55	55	49	48	49	51
85	55	55	52	54	46	45	46	47
80	53	52	52	52	44	43	44	46
75	51	50	50	50	42	41	42	45
70	50	49	49	48	40	40	41	42
65	48	48	48	47	39	39	40	40
60	47	46	47	45	38	38	38	39
55	46	45	46	44	37	37	37	37
50	45	44	45	43	35	36	36	36
45	43	43	44	42	34	35	35	35
40	42	42	43	41	33	33	34	34
35	41	41	41	41	32	32	33	33
30	40	40	40	40	31	31	31	31
25	39	39	39	39	30	30	30	30
20	37	36	37	37	29	29	30	29
15	36	35	35	36	27	27	28	26
10	34	33	33	34	25	25	25	25
5	30	30	30	31	21	22	22	21

From: American Alliance For Health, Physical Education, Recreation, and Dance: <u>Norms For College Students: Health Related Physical Fitness Test.</u> Reston, VA, 1985.

TEST COMPONENT #5 - UPPER BODY MUSCULAR STRENGTH

A. *Rationale*

While not a bona fide health-related fitness component, upper body strength (shoulders, chest, upper arms) is required for the performance of many sport, recreational, and occupational tasks. The 1-RM Bench Press measures the maximum weight pushed from the bench press position to full extension of the arms, and is used as a measure of upper body strength. The test is scored as a ratio of weight pushed, divided by your body weight.

B. Upper Body Muscular Strength Assessment: the 1-RM Bench Press Ratio Test

Equipment includes either a barbell set with a bench or a fixed bench press station on a single or multi-station apparatus. Determining the maximum weight you can lift in one repetition involves trial and error. Find a weight you can press two or three times. Add increments of 10 pounds and attempt the lift again. Add increments of 5 or 10 pounds (with rest between lifts) until you determine the maximum amount you can lift one time.

C. How Do You Rate on Upper Body Muscular Strength?

Compare your results with the normative standards in Table E-7 that have been developed in our university strength and conditioning classes.

Table E-7. Upper body bench press to body weight ratio norms [weight pushed (lb) divided by body weight (lb)]

Percentile	Female Age, y		Male Age, y	
	18-20	20-29	18-20	20-29
99	>0.90	>1.06	>1.70	>1.60
95	0.86	1.00	1.58	1.55
90	0.83	0.92	1.42	1.44
85	0.80	0.88	1.38	1.30
80	0.75	0.83	1.32	1.29
75	0.72	0.79	1.26	1.26
70	0.68	0.76	1.24	1.20
65	0.70	0.74	1.20	1.14
60	0.67	0.70	1.16	1.11
55	0.64	0.68	1.14	1.07
50	0.63	0.64	1.11	1.06
45	0.61	0.61	1.08	1.00
40	0.60	0.59	1.06	0.97
35	0.58	0.57	1.00	0.96
30	0.55	0.56	0.98	0.90
25	0.54	0.54	0.90	0.85
20	0.53	0.51	0.86	0.82
15	0.52	0.47	0.82	0.80
10	0.47	0.46	0.81	0.72
5	0.41	0.42	0.76	0.70
1	<0.39	<0.40	<0.68	>0.65

YOUR OVERALL HEALTH-RELATED FITNESS PROFILE

With a bar graph, visually display each component of your health-related fitness. Since scores on each item are not strongly related to each other (i.e., people with good muscular strength do not necessarily score high in aerobic fitness or flexibility, and vice versa), it is difficult for individuals to rank high on all items.

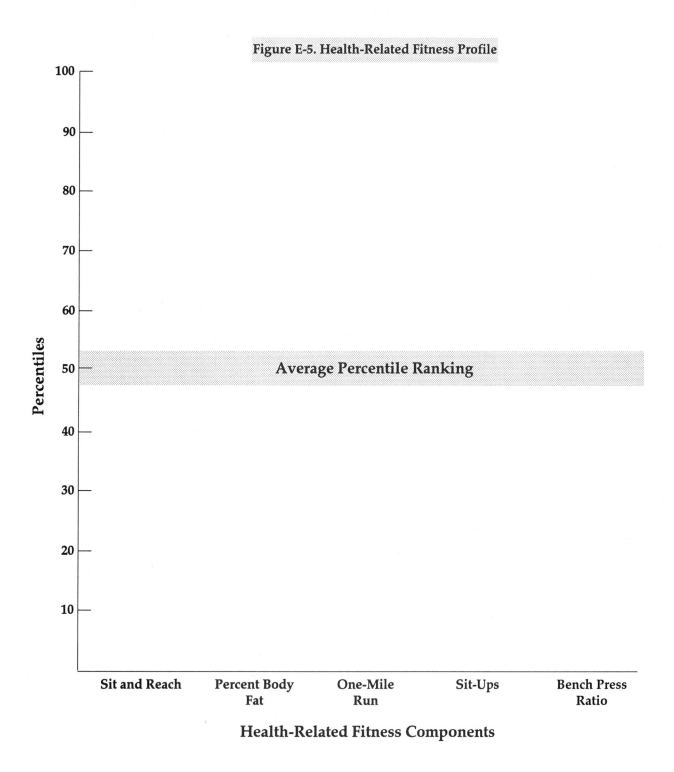

Figure E-5. Health-Related Fitness Profile

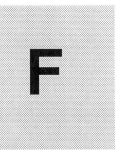

F ASSESSMENT OF HEART DISEASE RISK

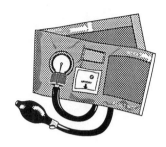

The assessment of heart disease risk factors will give you some idea of your chances of developing heart disease. The chart on the next page is a modified form of a more elaborate version generated from the more than 35 years of research on the natural history of heart disease in the community of Framingham, Massachusetts. The assessment is for adult men and women of all ages. While your heart disease risk score on is certainly not a substitute for a regular medical check-up, the information is helpful in providing insight as to potential areas for concern. Many of these telltale characteristics are habits or the result of habits that can be controlled. It certainly would be beneficial to identify risk factors at an early age (perhaps as young as two or three years!) to thwart the escalation of silent heart disease so prevalent in our highly mechanized, sedentary society.

Assign the appropriate numerical value that represents your present status for each category. Find the box applicable to you and circle the number in it. For example, if you are 19 years old, circle the number "1 pt" in the box labeled 10 to 20 years. After checking all the rows, add the circled numbers. The total number of points is your risk score. Refer to the **Relative Risk Category** to see how you rank. Keep in mind that there is nothing you can do about your age, gender, and heredity risk. Other risk factors such as high blood pressure, tension, cigarette smoking, serum cholesterol, diet, physical inactivity, and obesity can be modified, if not totally eliminated!

Explanation of Risk Variables

Heredity
Count parents, brothers, and sisters who have had a heart attack or stroke.

Smoking
If you inhale deeply and smoke a cigarette way down, add one point to your score. Do not subtract because you think you do not inhale or smoke only a half inch on a cigarette.

Exercise
Lower your score one point if you exercise regularly and frequently.

Cholesterol-Saturated Fat Intake
A cholesterol blood level is best. If you have not had a blood test recently, then estimate honestly the percentage of solid fats you eat. These are usually of animal origin like lard, cream, butter, and beef and lamb fat. If you eat much saturated fat, your cholesterol level will probably be high.

Blood Pressure
If you have no recent reading but have passed an insurance or general medical examination, chances are you have a systolic blood pressure level (upper reading) of 140 or less.

Gender
This takes into account the fact than men have from 6 to 10 times more heart attacks than women of child-bearing age.

	No known history of heart disease	1 relative with cardiovascular disease over age 60	2 relatives with cardiovascular disease over age 60	1 relative with cardiovascular disease under age 60	2 relatives with cardiovascular disease under age 60	3 relatives with cardiovascular disease under age 60
HEREDITY	1 pt	2 pts	3 pts	4 pts	6 pts	8 pts
AGE	10 to 20 1 pt	21 to 30 2 pts	31 to 40 3 pts	41 to 50 4 pts	51 to 60 6 pts	61 and over 8 pts
CHOLESTEROL OR DIETARY FAT%	Cholesterol below 180 mg/dl; diet contains no animal or solid fats 1 pt	Cholesterol 180-205 mg/dl; diet contains 10% animal or solid fats 2 pts	Cholesterol 206-230 mg/dl; diet contains 20% animal or solid fats 3 pts	Cholesterol 231-255 mg/dl; diet contains 30% animal or solid fats 4 pts	Cholesterol 256-280 mg/dl; diet contains 40% animal or solid fats 5 pts	Cholesterol 281-300 mg/dl; diet contains 50% animal or solid fats 7 pts
GENDER	Female under age 40 1 pt	Female age 40 to 50 2 pts	Female over age 50 3 pts	Male 4 pts	Stocky male 6 pts	Bald stocky male 7 pts
EXERCISE	Intensive occupational and recreational exertion 1 pt	Moderate occupational and recreational exertion 2 pts	Sedentary work and intense recreational exertion 3 pts	Sedentary occupational and moderate recreational exertion 5 pts	Sedentary work and light recreational exertion 6 pts	Complete lack of all exercise 3 pts
BLOOD PRESSURE	100 upper reading 1 pt	120 upper reading 2 pts	140 upper reading 3 pts	160 upper reading 4 pts	180 upper reading 6 pts	200 or more upper reading 8 pts
TOBACCO SMOKING	Non-user 0 pts	Cigar and/or pipe 1 pt	10 cigarettes or less per day 3 pts	20 cigarettes per day 4 pts	30 cigarettes per day 6 pts	40 cigarettes per day 8 pts
BODY WEIGHT	+5 lbs below standard weight 0 pts	-5 to +5 lbs of standard weight 1 pt	6 to 20 lbs over weight 2 pts	21 to 35 lbs over weight 3 pts	36 to 50 lbs over weight 5 pts	51 to 65 lbs over weight 7 pts

SCORE	RELATIVE RISK CATEGORY	SCORE	RELATIVE RISK CATEGORY
6 to 11	Risk well below average	25 to 31	Moderate risk
12 to 17	Risk below average	32 to 40	High risk
18 to 24	Average risk	41 to 62	Very high risk, see a doctor

SECTION III

- **ANSWERS TO CHAPTER QUIZZES**

- **CROSSWORD PUZZLE SOLUTIONS**

- **TIPS ON PREPARING FOR EXAMS**

PART A

ANSWERS TO CHAPTER QUIZZES

Chapter 1 (p. 35)

Multiple Choice	Fill-In	True/False
1. c	1. 11	1. F
2. b	2. RNA	2. F
3. b	3. ions	3. T
4. a	4. respiration	4. F
5. b	5. loses; gains	5. F

Chapter 2 (p. 24)

Multiple Choice	Fill-In	True/False
1. a	1. hepatic-portal vein	1. F
2. a	2. pyloric sphincter	2. F
3. a	3. villi	3. F
4. d	4. lacteals	4. T
5. b	5. bile	5. F

Chapter 3 (p. 35)

Multiple Choice	Fill-In	True/False
1. a	1. glucose, fructose, galactose	1. F
2. e	2. lactose	2. F
3. e	3. water-soluble	3. T
4. d	4. gluconeogenesis	4. F
5. c	5. glucagon	5. T

Chapter 4 (p. 47)

Multiple Choice	Fill-In	True/False
1. d	1. unsaturated	1. F
2. a	2. triglyceride	2. T
3. e	3. polyunsaturated	3. F
4. e	4. 9	4. F
5. e	5. 30	5. T

Chapter 5 (p. 57)

Multiple Choice	Fill-In	True/False
1. b	1. 100	1. F
2. e	2. peptide bonds	2. T
3. e	3. deamination	3. T
4. e	4. nutritent density	4. T
5. d	5. lactovegetarian	5. T

Chapter 6 (p. 65)

Multiple Choice	Fill-In	True/False
1. d	1. ascorbic acid	1. F
2. b	2. 50	2. T
3. b	3. 10	3. F
4. a	4. thirteen	4. F
5. a	5. vitamin B_{12}	5. F

Chapter 7 (p. 75)

Multiple Choice	Fill-In	True/False
1. e	1. milk, cheese, legumes, green vegetables	1. T
2. b	2. electrolytes	2. F
3. b	3. goiter	3. T
4. e	4. hydroxyapatite	4. T
5. e	5. osteoporosis	5. T

Chapter 8 (p. 82)

Multiple Choice	Fill-In	True/False
1. d	1. diabetes	1. F
2. c	2. insensible	2. T
3. b	3. sweat	3. T
4. c	4. relative humidity	4. F
5. b	5. hyperthermia	5. F

Chapter 9 (p. 90)

Multiple Choice	Fill-In	True/False
1. d	1. 60-70	1. T
2. b	2. fortified	2. F
3. a	3. GRAS	3. T
4. e	4. low calorie, reduced calorie	4. F
5. d	5. Bureau of Alcohol Tobacco, and Firearms	5. T

Chapter 10 (p. 99)

Multiple Choice	Fill-In	True/False
1. b	1. 0.8	1. T
2. b	2. 30	2. F
3. d	3. 60	3. T
4. c	4. fat	4. T
5. d	5. hitting the wall	5. F

Chapter 11 (p. 112)

Multiple Choice	Fill-In	True/False
1. e	1. ATP	1. F
2. b	2. phosphate	2. F
3. b	3. glycolysis	3. T
4. b	4. hydrogen	4. F
5. a	5. max VO2	5. T

Chapter 12 (p. 124)

Multiple Choice	Fill-In	True/False
1. c	1. alveoli	1. T
2. a	2. diaphragm	2. T
3. a	3. diffusion	3. F
4. a	4. capillaries	4. F
5. a	5. 120	5. T

Chapter 13 (p. 132)

Multiple Choice	Fill-In	True/False
1. a	1. protein	1. F
2. b	2. 1.7	2. F
3. a	3. increase	3. F
4. b	4. open-circuit	4. F
5. d	5. resting, thermogenesis physical activity	5. T

Chapter 14 (p. 147)

Multiple Choice	Fill-In	True/False
1. d	1. residual lung volume	1. F
2. e	2. hydrostatic weighing	2. F
3. c	3. underestimate	3. T
4. c	4. body volume	4. F
5. a	5. 13% to 17%	5. F

Chapter 15 (p. 156)

Multiple Choice	Fill-In	True/False
1. e	1. three	1. T
2. c	2. 30	2. T
3. e	3. lipoprotein lipase	3. F
4. a	4. adipocytes	4. F
5. d	5. hypertrophy	5. T

Chapter 16 (p. 167)

Multiple Choice	Fill-In	True/False
1. b	1. diet, exercise, diet+exer	1. T
2. e	2. 5%	2. T
3. d	3. one	3. T
4. d	4. muscle (lean); fat	4. T
5. d	5. carbohydrate, water	5. T

Chapter 17 (p. 175)

Multiple Choice	Fill-In	True/False
1. d	1. daily exercise	1. T
2. c	2. behavior modification	2. T
3. b	3. bulemia nervosa	3. F
4. d	4. less	4. T
5. a	5. pedometers	5. T

Chapter 19 (p. 200)

Multiple Choice	Fill-In	True/False
1. e	1. intensity	1. F
2. b	2. anaerobic	2. F
3. d	3. 8	3. F
4. f	4. 70	4. T
5. e	5. exercise duration	5. F

Chapter 18 (p. 187)

Multiple Choice	Fill-In	True/False
1. e	1. Fast	1. T
2. b	2. 50	2. F
3. e	3. circuit resistance training	3. T
4. a	4. isokinetic training	4. F
5. d	5. neural	5. F

Chapter 20 (p. 214)

Multiple Choice	Fill-In	True/False
1. b	1. 170	1. T
2. c	2. 2000	2. F
3. e	3. heart attack	3. T
4. e	4. coronary circulation	4. F
5. b	5. atherosclerosis	5. T

PART B

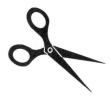

CROSSWORD PUZZLE SOLUTIONS

Chapter 1

Across and down solutions include: BUFFER, IONIC BOND, PEPTIDE, CHEMICAL, BASE, BULK, ELECTRON, ELEMENTS, ENERGY, MATTER, ORGAN, ATOMS, IONS, ACIDS, KINETIC, LOCK, COLLOID, ACIDOSIS, BIOLOGIC WORK

Chapter 2

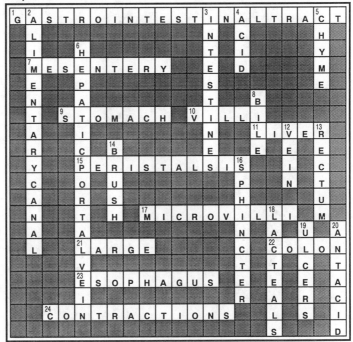

Across and down solutions include: GASTROINTESTINAL TRACT, MESENTERY, STOMACH, VILLI, LIVER, PERISTALSIS, MICROVILLI, LARGE, COLON, ESOPHAGUS, CONTRACTIONS

CROSSWORD PUZZLE SOLUTIONS

Chapter 3

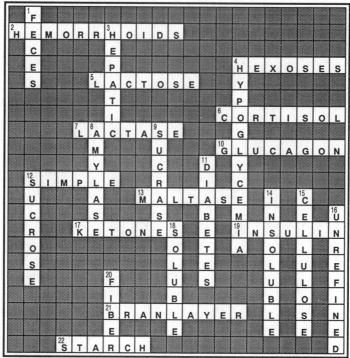

Chapter 4

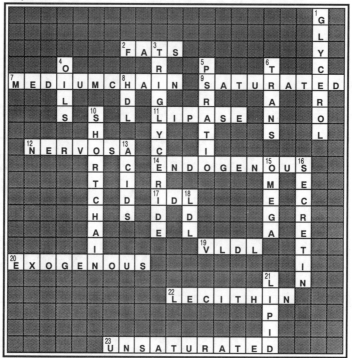

CROSSWORD PUZZLE SOLUTIONS

Chapter 5

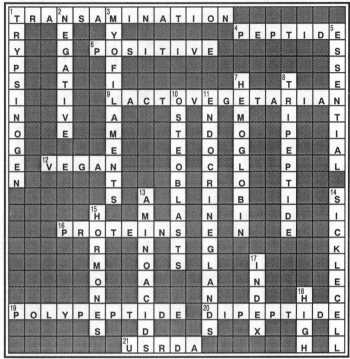

Chapter 6

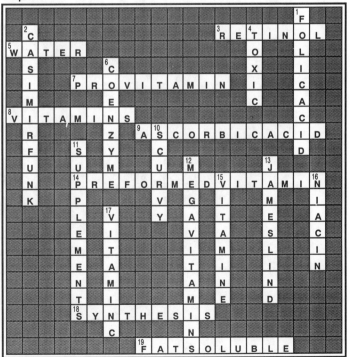

CROSSWORD PUZZLE SOLUTIONS

Chapter 7

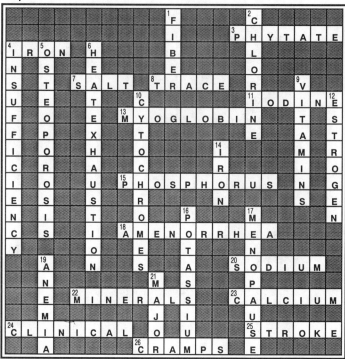

Chapter 8

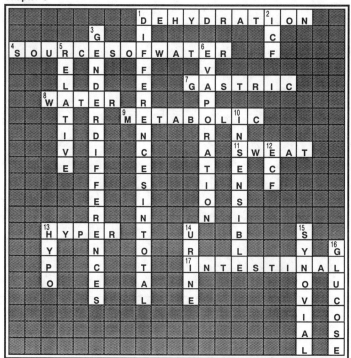

CROSSWORD PUZZLE SOLUTIONS

Chapter 9

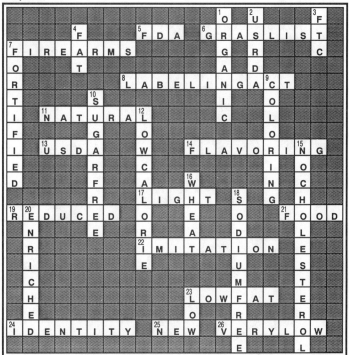

Chapter 10

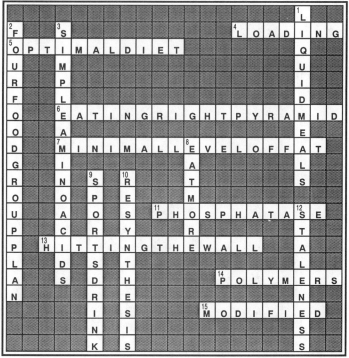

CROSSWORD PUZZLE SOLUTIONS

Chapter 11

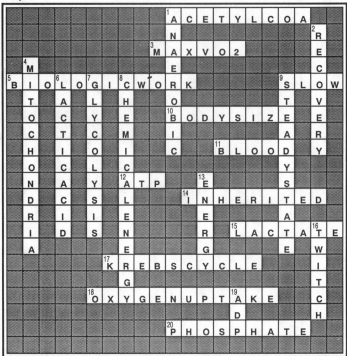

Chapter 12

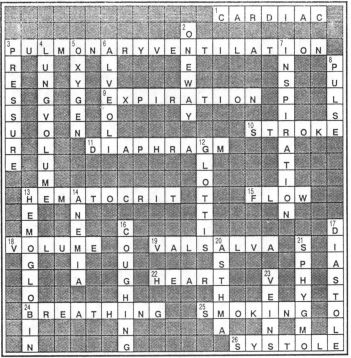

CROSSWORD PUZZLE SOLUTIONS

Chapter 13

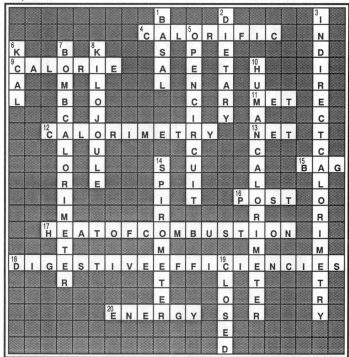

Chapter 14

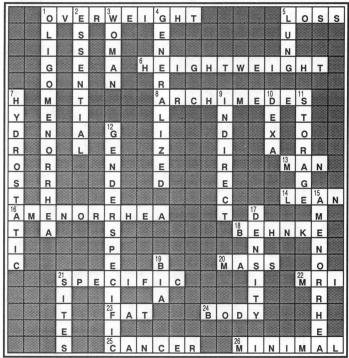

CROSSWORD PUZZLE SOLUTIONS

Chapter 15

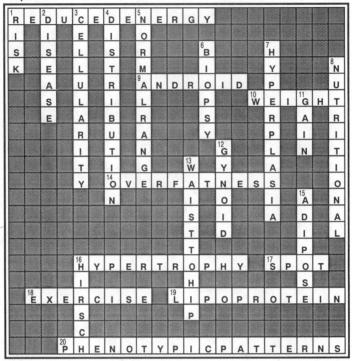

Chapter 16

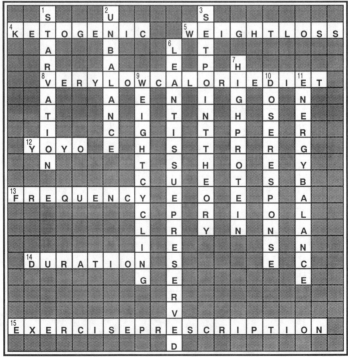

CROSSWORD PUZZLE SOLUTIONS

Chapter 17

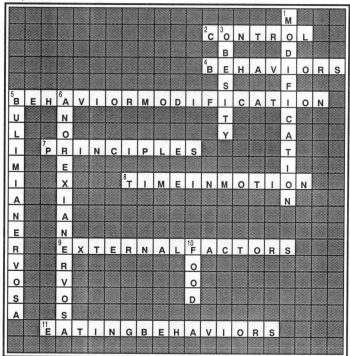

Chapter 18

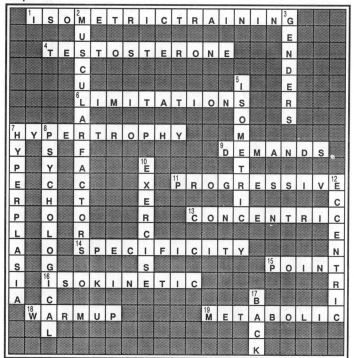

CROSSWORD PUZZLE SOLUTIONS

Chapter 19

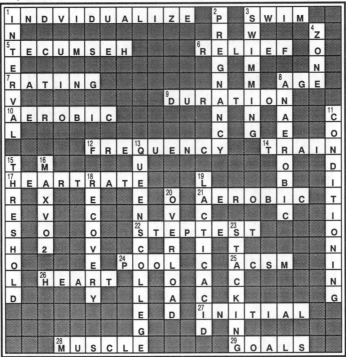

Chapter 20

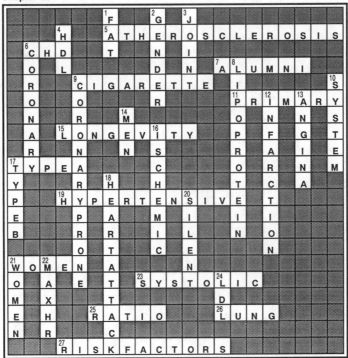

PART C

TIPS ON PREPARING FOR EXAMS

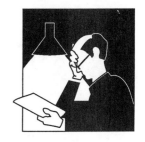

Proper Planning Prevents Poor Performance

From our experience as college students, we know the trauma and uncertainty that precedes exams. We know first-hand how difficult it is to feel adequately prepared to take an exam, and we must admit, we too were not always successful. But we never gave up, and over the years both as students and now as professors, we have gained respect for proper planning. Below are three principles or "tips" that will help prepare you to take any exam, and prevent poor performance.

1. Preparation Principle. Begin the review process at least seven days before the exam. Unless you have a photographic memory, fewer days of preparation are probably inadequate. The common practice of late night cramming is only slightly better for one's overall psyche and health than walking blindfolded down the center lane of a highway! Although many students still "cram" all night for exams, the end result is usually the same - "I could have done better if only I had more tome to study!" With even a modicum of planning, you can avoid that nighttime walk down the highway, and you'll feel better too, especially when you get your grade. To those who don't heed the advise - well, at least we tried to warn you.

2. Concentration Principle. Intensity of effort yields a higher return, to use a financial metaphor, than duration of effort. Translation: It's not how many hours you devote to note taking, underlining, or reviewing, but it's how much you concentrate when you do study that really counts. Here's a tip to help you concentrate. For text reading, instead of underlining with a colored marker, read two or three lines of text, and then cover up the section and repeat out loud what you just read. Sounds easy? Try it! You'll find that this simple task is very challenging. Don't give up if at first you have trouble. Try again, and again. Really concentrate on what you read, and then verbalize it immediately. **The verbalization is crucial.** For those able to concentrate, you should have little problem reciting back the key elements or salient points.

If you have difficulty with this exercise, don't be discouraged. Reading with concentration is not an easy task. It is something that must be learned. And as in learning any new skill, gratification does not come immediately. If you're a golfer or tennis player, you know what we mean (especially the golfers!).

Through experience, we have found that this **read-and-recite** method can improve comprehension by as much as 85%! As you become more proficient, you'll be able to recite more facts and concepts. And once you truly have learned something, recalling and remembering for exams should be a piece of cake!

3. Perfect Practice Principle. The saying is commonplace, "Practice makes perfect." Right? Wrong! We would change the sentence to read, "**Perfect practice makes perfect.**" What do we mean? Suppose you practiced incorrectly. The more you practiced, the better you would become at doing it wrong! Now that really would be counterproductive and a great waste of your time and effort.

We suggest that you consider in advance what types of questions will be asked and then practice getting the answers to similar questions. We realize this is sometimes difficult, but here are a few hints. If you know in advance that the questions were going to be multiple choice, the application of the perfect practice principle would be to practice using multiple choice questions. It's that simple. In fact, it would be helpful to design your own multiple choice questions. You'll be surprised how easy it is to do, and how much it helps you prepare for an exam.

Important Dates

Assignment Due Dates:

Assignment #1 _____

Assignment #2 _____

Assignment #3 _____

Assignment #4 _____

Assignment #5 _____

Assignment #6 _____

Assignment #7 _____

Assignment #8 _____

Assignment #9 _____

Exam Dates:

Exam #1 _____

Exam #1 _____

Exam #1 _____

Mid-term _____

Mid-term _____

Final exam _____

Holiday Dates:

1. _____

2. _____

3. _____

4. _____

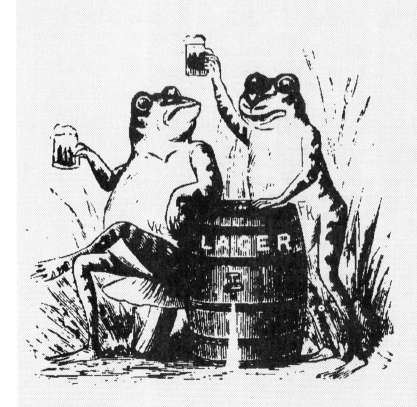

1993

JANUARY
S	M	T	W	T	F	S
					1	2
3	4	5	6	7	8	9
10	11	12	13	14	15	16
17	18	19	20	21	22	23
24	25	26	27	28	29	30
31						

MARCH
S	M	T	W	T	F	S
	1	2	3	4	5	6
7	8	9	10	11	12	13
14	15	16	17	18	19	20
21	22	23	24	25	26	27
28	29	30	31			

MAY
S	M	T	W	T	F	S
						1
2	3	4	5	6	7	8
9	10	11	12	13	14	15
16	17	18	19	20	21	22
23	24	25	26	27	28	29
30	31					

JULY
S	M	T	W	T	F	S
				1	2	3
4	5	6	7	8	9	10
11	12	13	14	15	16	17
18	19	20	21	22	23	24
25	26	27	28	29	30	31

SEPTEMBER
S	M	T	W	T	F	S
			1	2	3	4
5	6	7	8	9	10	11
12	13	14	15	16	17	18
19	20	21	22	23	24	25
26	27	28	29	30		

NOVEMBER
S	M	T	W	T	F	S
	1	2	3	4	5	6
7	8	9	10	11	12	13
14	15	16	17	18	19	20
21	22	23	24	25	26	27
28	29	30				

IMPORTANT DATES

JANUARY
1 New Year's Day
18 Martin Luther King's Birthday (Observed)
FEBRUARY
12 Lincoln's Birthday
14 Valentine's Day
15 Washington's Birthday (Observed)
24 Ash Wednesday
MARCH
17 St. Patrick's Day
21 Mothering Sunday (U.K.)
APRIL
4 Daylight Saving Time Begins
4 Palm Sunday
6 First Day of Passover
9 Good Friday
11 Easter
12 Easter Monday (Canada)
MAY
3 May Day Holiday (U.K.)
9 Mother's Day
15 Armed Forces Day
24 Victoria Day (Canada)
31 Memorial Day
31 Spring Holiday (U.K. not Scotland)
JUNE
7 Holiday (Republic of Ireland)
14 Flag Day
20 Father's Day
JULY
1 Canada Day
4 Independence Day
12 Holiday (N. Ireland)
AUGUST
2 Holiday (Republic of Ireland)
30 Late Summer Holiday (U.K. not Scotland)
SEPTEMBER
6 Labor Day
16 First Day of Rosh Hashanah
25 Yom Kippur
OCTOBER
11 Columbus Day
11 Thanksgiving Day (Canada)
31 Daylight Saving Time Ends
31 Halloween
NOVEMBER
2 Election Day
11 Veterans Day
11 Remembrance Day (Canada)
25 Thanksgiving Day
DECEMBER
9 First Day of Hanukkah
25 Christmas
27 Boxing Day

FEBRUARY
S	M	T	W	T	F	S
	1	2	3	4	5	6
7	8	9	10	11	12	13
14	15	16	17	18	19	20
21	22	23	24	25	26	27
28						

APRIL
S	M	T	W	T	F	S
				1	2	3
4	5	6	7	8	9	10
11	12	13	14	15	16	17
18	19	20	21	22	23	24
25	26	27	28	29	30	

JUNE
S	M	T	W	T	F	S
		1	2	3	4	5
6	7	8	9	10	11	12
13	14	15	16	17	18	19
20	21	22	23	24	25	26
27	28	29	30			

AUGUST
S	M	T	W	T	F	S
1	2	3	4	5	6	7
8	9	10	11	12	13	14
15	16	17	18	19	20	21
22	23	24	25	26	27	28
29	30	31				

OCTOBER
S	M	T	W	T	F	S
					1	2
3	4	5	6	7	8	9
10	11	12	13	14	15	16
17	18	19	20	21	22	23
24	25	26	27	28	29	30
31						

DECEMBER
S	M	T	W	T	F	S
			1	2	3	4
5	6	7	8	9	10	11
12	13	14	15	16	17	18
19	20	21	22	23	24	25
26	27	28	29	30	31	

1994

JANUARY
S	M	T	W	T	F	S
						1
2	3	4	5	6	7	8
9	10	11	12	13	14	15
16	17	18	19	20	21	22
23	24	25	26	27	28	29
30	31					

MARCH
S	M	T	W	T	F	S
		1	2	3	4	5
6	7	8	9	10	11	12
13	14	15	16	17	18	19
20	21	22	23	24	25	26
27	28	29	30	31		

MAY
S	M	T	W	T	F	S
1	2	3	4	5	6	7
8	9	10	11	12	13	14
15	16	17	18	19	20	21
22	23	24	25	26	27	28
29	30	31				

JULY
S	M	T	W	T	F	S
					1	2
3	4	5	6	7	8	9
10	11	12	13	14	15	16
17	18	19	20	21	22	23
24	25	26	27	28	29	30
31						

SEPTEMBER
S	M	T	W	T	F	S
				1	2	3
4	5	6	7	8	9	10
11	12	13	14	15	16	17
18	19	20	21	22	23	24
25	26	27	28	29	30	

NOVEMBER
S	M	T	W	T	F	S
		1	2	3	4	5
6	7	8	9	10	11	12
13	14	15	16	17	18	19
20	21	22	23	24	25	26
27	28	29	30			

IMPORTANT DATES

JANUARY
1 New Year's Day
17 Martin Luther King's Birthday (Observed)
FEBRUARY
12 Lincoln's Birthday
14 Valentine's Day
16 Ash Wednesday
21 Washington's Birthday (Observed)
MARCH
13 Mothering Sunday (U.K.)
17 St. Patrick's Day
27 Palm Sunday
27 First Day of Passover
APRIL
1 Good Friday
3 Daylight Saving Time Begins
3 Easter
4 Easter Monday (Canada)
MAY
2 May Day Holiday (U.K.)
8 Mother's Day
21 Armed Forces Day
23 Victoria Day (Canada)
30 Memorial Day
30 Spring Holiday (U.K. not Scotland)
JUNE
6 Holiday (Republic of Ireland)
14 Flag Day
19 Father's Day
JULY
1 Canada Day
4 Independence Day
12 Holiday (N. Ireland)
AUGUST
1 Holiday (Republic of Ireland)
29 Late Summer Holiday (U.K. not Scotland)
SEPTEMBER
5 Labor Day
6 First Day of Rosh Hashanah
15 Yom Kippur
OCTOBER
10 Columbus Day
10 Thanksgiving Day (Canada)
30 Daylight Saving Time Ends
31 Halloween
NOVEMBER
8 Election Day
11 Veterans Day
11 Remembrance Day (Canada)
24 Thanksgiving Day
28 First Day of Hanukkah
DECEMBER
25 Christmas
26 Boxing Day

FEBRUARY
S	M	T	W	T	F	S
		1	2	3	4	5
6	7	8	9	10	11	12
13	14	15	16	17	18	19
20	21	22	23	24	25	26
27	28					

APRIL
S	M	T	W	T	F	S
					1	2
3	4	5	6	7	8	9
10	11	12	13	14	15	16
17	18	19	20	21	22	23
24	25	26	27	28	29	30

JUNE
S	M	T	W	T	F	S
			1	2	3	4
5	6	7	8	9	10	11
12	13	14	15	16	17	18
19	20	21	22	23	24	25
26	27	28	29	30		

AUGUST
S	M	T	W	T	F	S
	1	2	3	4	5	6
7	8	9	10	11	12	13
14	15	16	17	18	19	20
21	22	23	24	25	26	27
28	29	30	31			

OCTOBER
S	M	T	W	T	F	S
						1
2	3	4	5	6	7	8
9	10	11	12	13	14	15
16	17	18	19	20	21	22
23	24	25	26	27	28	29
30	31					

DECEMBER
S	M	T	W	T	F	S
				1	2	3
4	5	6	7	8	9	10
11	12	13	14	15	16	17
18	19	20	21	22	23	24
25	26	27	28	29	30	31

1995

JANUARY
```
S  M  T  W  T  F  S
1  2  3  4  5  6  7
8  9 10 11 12 13 14
15 16 17 18 19 20 21
22 23 24 25 26 27 28
29 30 31
```

MARCH
```
S  M  T  W  T  F  S
         1  2  3  4
5  6  7  8  9 10 11
12 13 14 15 16 17 18
19 20 21 22 23 24 25
26 27 28 29 30 31
```

MAY
```
S  M  T  W  T  F  S
1  2  3  4  5  6
7  8  9 10 11 12 13
14 15 16 17 18 19 20
21 22 23 24 25 26 27
28 29 30 31
```

JULY
```
S  M  T  W  T  F  S
                  1
2  3  4  5  6  7  8
9 10 11 12 13 14 15
16 17 18 19 20 21 22
23 24 25 26 27 28 29
30 31
```

SEPTEMBER
```
S  M  T  W  T  F  S
                1  2
3  4  5  6  7  8  9
10 11 12 13 14 15 16
17 18 19 20 21 22 23
24 25 26 27 28 29 30
```

NOVEMBER
```
S  M  T  W  T  F  S
         1  2  3  4
5  6  7  8  9 10 11
12 13 14 15 16 17 18
19 20 21 22 23 24 25
26 27 28 29 30
```

IMPORTANT DATES

JANUARY
1 New Year's Day
16 Martin Luther King's Birthday
   (Observed)

FEBRUARY
12 Lincoln's Birthday
14 Valentine's Day
20 Washington's Birthday (Observed)

MARCH
1 Ash Wednesday
17 St. Patrick's Day
26 Mothering Sunday (U.K.)

APRIL
2 Daylight Saving Time Begins
9 Palm Sunday
14 Good Friday
15 First Day of Passover
16 Easter
17 Easter Monday (Canada)

MAY
1 May Day Holiday (U.K.)
14 Mother's Day
20 Armed Forces Day
22 Victoria Day (Canada)
29 Memorial Day
29 Spring Holiday
   (U.K. not Scotland)

JUNE
5 Holiday (Republic of Ireland)
14 Flag Day
18 Father's Day

JULY
1 Canada Day
4 Independence Day
12 Holiday (N. Ireland)

AUGUST
7 Holiday (Republic of Ireland)
28 Late Summer Holiday
   (U.K. not Scotland)

SEPTEMBER
4 Labor Day
25 First Day of Rosh Hashanah

OCTOBER
4 Yom Kippur
9 Columbus Day
9 Thanksgiving Day (Canada)
29 Daylight Saving Time Ends
31 Halloween

NOVEMBER
7 Election Day
11 Veterans Day
11 Remembrance Day (Canada)
23 Thanksgiving Day

DECEMBER
18 First Day of Hanukkah
25 Christmas

FEBRUARY
```
S  M  T  W  T  F  S
            1  2  3  4
5  6  7  8  9 10 11
12 13 14 15 16 17 18
19 20 21 22 23 24 25
26 27 28
```

APRIL
```
S  M  T  W  T  F  S
                  1
2  3  4  5  6  7  8
9 10 11 12 13 14 15
16 17 18 19 20 21 22
23 24 25 26 27 28 29
30
```

JUNE
```
S  M  T  W  T  F  S
            1  2  3
4  5  6  7  8  9 10
11 12 13 14 15 16 17
18 19 20 21 22 23 24
25 26 27 28 29 30
```

AUGUST
```
S  M  T  W  T  F  S
      1  2  3  4  5
6  7  8  9 10 11 12
13 14 15 16 17 18 19
20 21 22 23 24 25 26
27 28 29 30 31
```

OCTOBER
```
S  M  T  W  T  F  S
1  2  3  4  5  6  7
8  9 10 11 12 13 14
15 16 17 18 19 20 21
22 23 24 25 26 27 28
29 30 31
```

DECEMBER
```
S  M  T  W  T  F  S
                  1  2
3  4  5  6  7  8  9
10 11 12 13 14 15 16
17 18 19 20 21 22 23
24 25 26 27 28 29 30
```

1996

JANUARY
```
S  M  T  W  T  F  S
1  2  3  4  5  6
7  8  9 10 11 12 13
14 15 16 17 18 19 20
21 22 23 24 25 26 27
28 29 30 31
```

MARCH
```
S  M  T  W  T  F  S
               1  2
3  4  5  6  7  8  9
10 11 12 13 14 15 16
17 18 19 20 21 22 23
24 25 26 27 28 29 30
31
```

MAY
```
S  M  T  W  T  F  S
         1  2  3  4
5  6  7  8  9 10 11
12 13 14 15 16 17 18
19 20 21 22 23 24 25
26 27 28 29 30 31
```

JULY
```
S  M  T  W  T  F  S
1  2  3  4  5  6
7  8  9 10 11 12 13
14 15 16 17 18 19 20
21 22 23 24 25 26 27
28 29 30 31
```

SEPTEMBER
```
S  M  T  W  T  F  S
1  2  3  4  5  6  7
8  9 10 11 12 13 14
15 16 17 18 19 20 21
22 23 24 25 26 27 28
29 30
```

NOVEMBER
```
S  M  T  W  T  F  S
                  1  2
3  4  5  6  7  8  9
10 11 12 13 14 15 16
17 18 19 20 21 22 23
24 25 26 27 28 29 30
```

IMPORTANT DATES

JANUARY
1 New Year's Day
15 Martin Luther King's Birthday
   (Observed)

FEBRUARY
12 Lincoln's Birthday
14 Valentine's Day
19 Washington's Birthday (Observed)
21 Ash Wednesday

MARCH
17 St. Patrick's Day
17 Mothering Sunday (U.K.)
31 Palm Sunday

APRIL
4 First Day of Passover
5 Good Friday
7 Easter
7 Daylight Saving Time Begins
8 Easter Monday (Canada)

MAY
6 May Day Holiday (U.K.)
12 Mother's Day
18 Armed Forces Day
20 Victoria Day (Canada)
27 Memorial Day
27 Spring Holiday
   (U.K. not Scotland)

JUNE
3 Holiday (Republic of Ireland)
14 Flag Day
16 Father's Day

JULY
1 Canada Day
4 Independence Day
12 Holiday (N. Ireland)

AUGUST
5 Holiday (Republic of Ireland)
26 Late Summer Holiday
   (U.K. not Scotland)

SEPTEMBER
2 Labor Day
14 First Day of Rosh Hashanah
23 Yom Kippur

OCTOBER
14 Columbus Day
14 Thanksgiving Day (Canada)
27 Daylight Saving Time Ends
31 Halloween

NOVEMBER
5 Election Day
11 Veterans Day
11 Remembrance Day (Canada)
28 Thanksgiving Day

DECEMBER
6 First Day of Hanukkah
25 Christmas
26 Boxing Day

FEBRUARY
```
S  M  T  W  T  F  S
            1  2  3
4  5  6  7  8  9 10
11 12 13 14 15 16 17
18 19 20 21 22 23 24
25 26 27 28 29
```

APRIL
```
S  M  T  W  T  F  S
1  2  3  4  5  6
7  8  9 10 11 12 13
14 15 16 17 18 19 20
21 22 23 24 25 26 27
28 29 30
```

JUNE
```
S  M  T  W  T  F  S
                  1
2  3  4  5  6  7  8
9 10 11 12 13 14 15
16 17 18 19 20 21 22
23 24 25 26 27 28 29
30
```

AUGUST
```
S  M  T  W  T  F  S
            1  2  3
4  5  6  7  8  9 10
11 12 13 14 15 16 17
18 19 20 21 22 23 24
25 26 27 28 29 30 31
```

OCTOBER
```
S  M  T  W  T  F  S
         1  2  3  4  5
6  7  8  9 10 11 12
13 14 15 16 17 18 19
20 21 22 23 24 25 26
27 28 29 30 31
```

DECEMBER
```
S  M  T  W  T  F  S
1  2  3  4  5  6  7
8  9 10 11 12 13 14
15 16 17 18 19 20 21
22 23 24 25 26 27 28
29 30 31
```

Notes

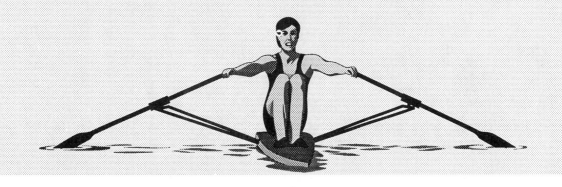

Notes

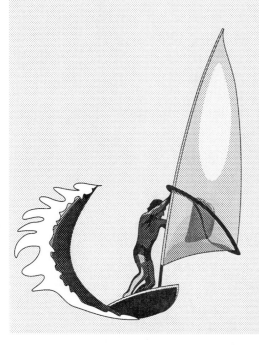

Notes

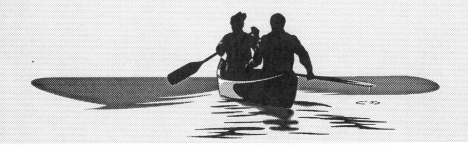

Notes

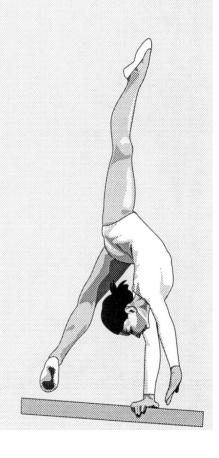

Notes

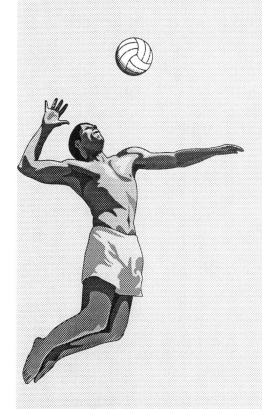

Notes

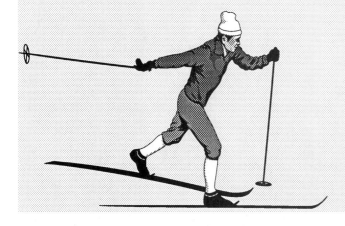